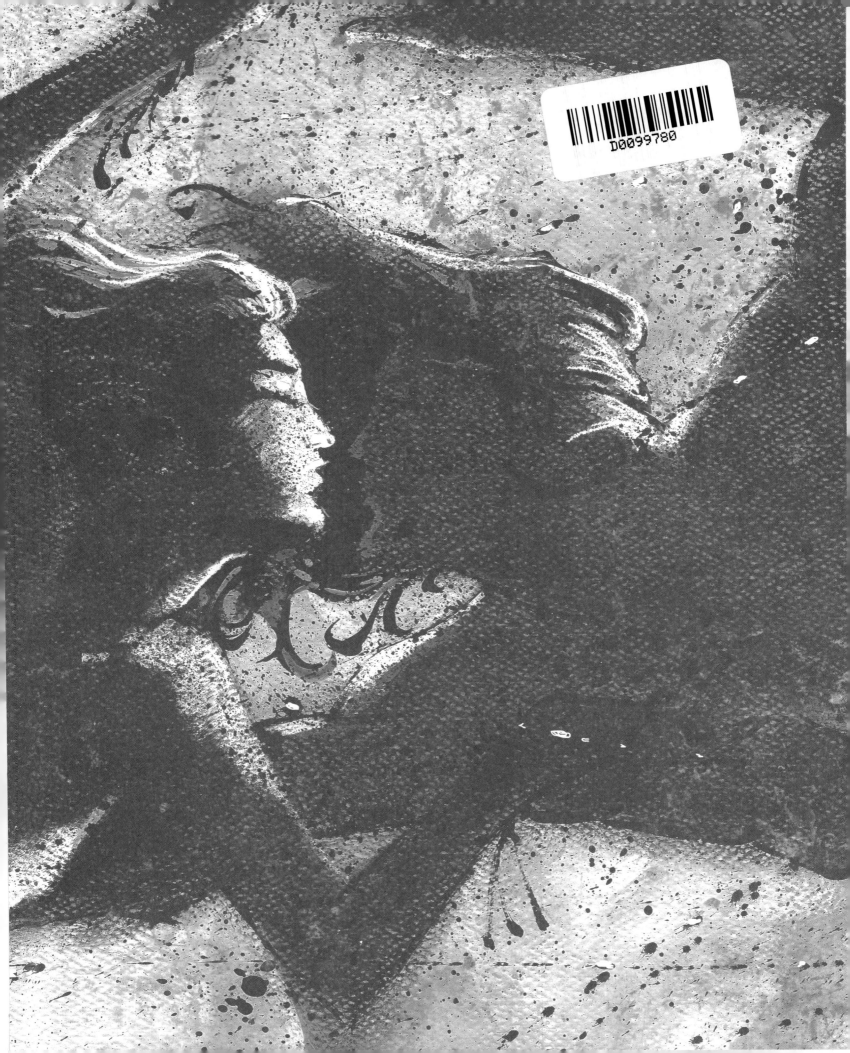

First published in the United States and Great Britain in 2006 by

Virgin Books Ltd
Thames Wharf Studios
Rainville Road
London
W6 9HA

A catalogue record for this book is available from the British Library.

ISBN 1 85227 385 2
ISBN 9 781852 273859

The paper used in this book is a natural, recyclable product made from wood grown in sustainable forests. The manufacturing process conforms to the regulations of the country of origin.

Book art direction and design by Mystery.co.uk

Printed and bound by Rotolito Lombarda

CONTENTS

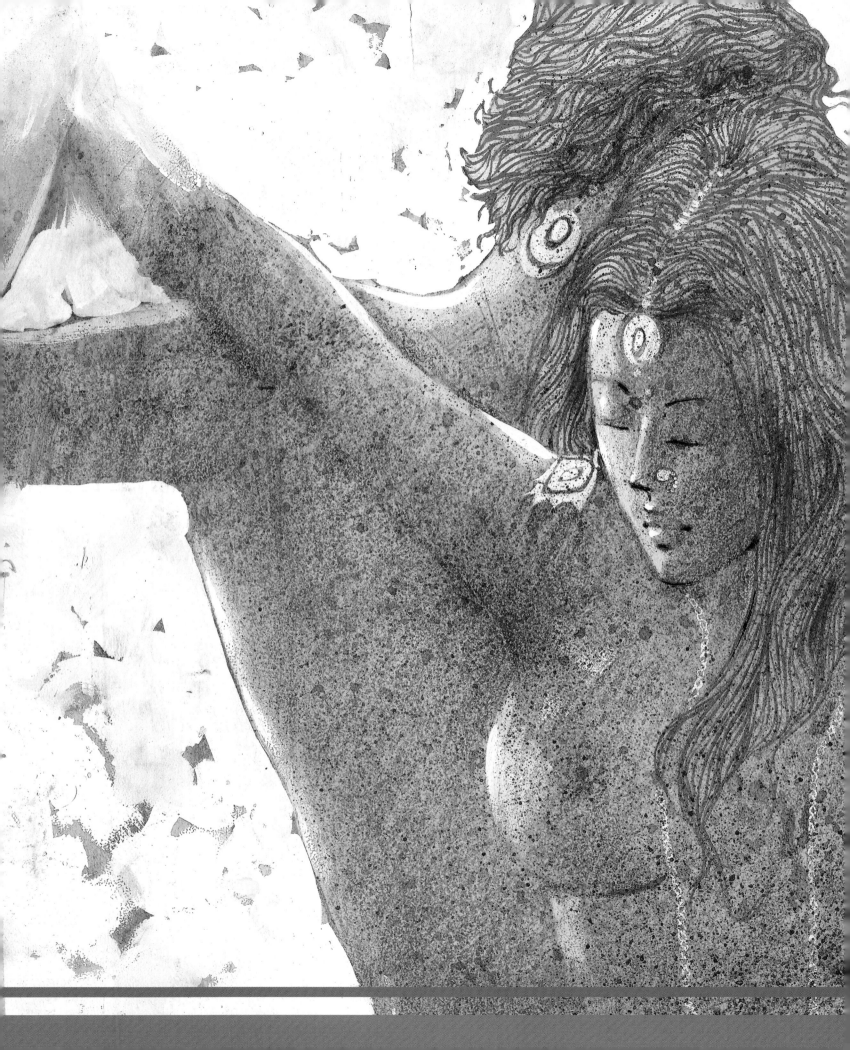

PREFACE

In the interest of authenticity I decided to retain certain aspects of the original **Kama Sutra** *that reflect the biases and prejudices of an ancient culture (references to Lepers, Women of Caste, certain complexions etc). If anything these crude sections serve as a reminder of how far we have come in our awareness, how long it has taken to get here, and how far we still have to go. The* **Kama Sutra** *is timeless in its depth and understanding of eroticism. Yet as time marches on and our attitudes and understanding of self evolve, certain aspects of the* **Kama Sutra** *become irrelevant and fossils of a time gone by. The contemporary reader is asked to read the* **Kama Sutra** *keeping in mind its historical context while relating to its essence.*

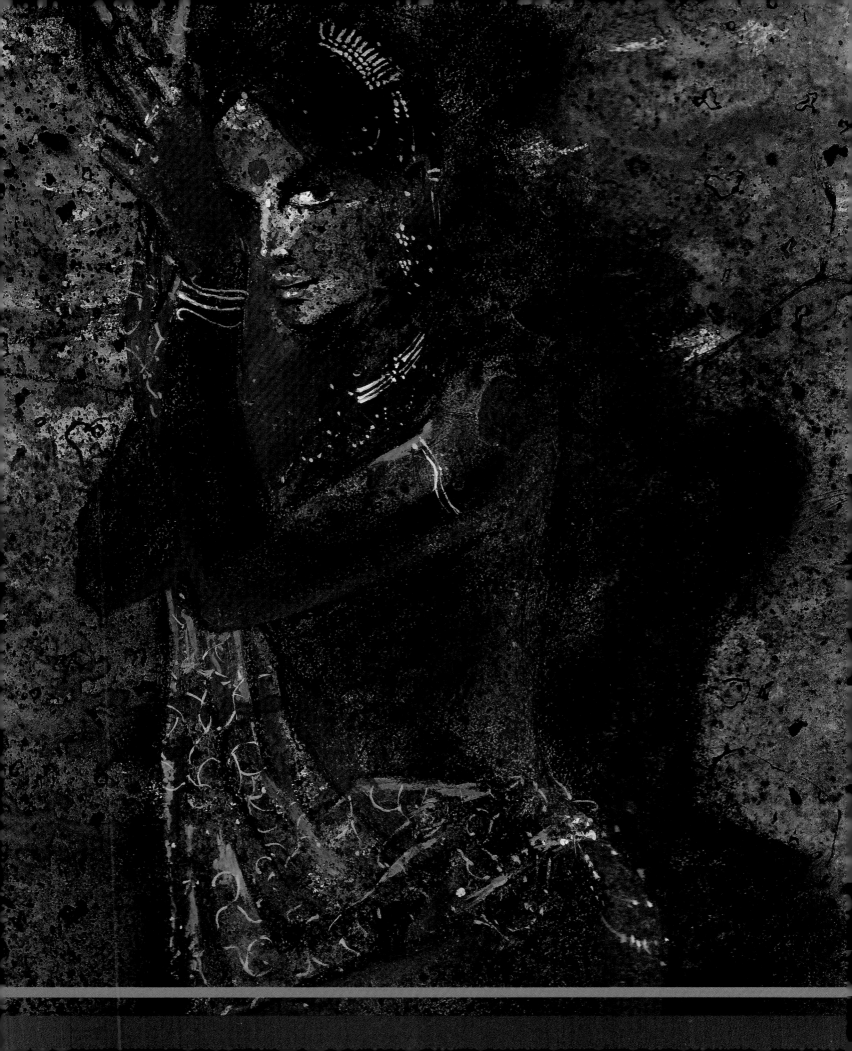

CHAPTER 1

DELIGHT & THE SOUL

*T*he Kama Sutra *is many things: a manual for lovemaking, a venerable ancient text of India, a marital aid sneaked furtively into many a bedroom and, to prudes throughout the ages, a scandal.*

Can it also be described as an inspiring spiritual text?

I strongly believe it can. In the West sex and spirit have been tragically divorced. Although the Old Testament contains marriage customs that would be titillating or socially unacceptable today, particularly polygamy, the New Testament brought down a curtain of shame over sex that still weighs heavy.

We may not agree with Saint Paul that 'it is better to marry than to burn', a phrase which assumes that sexual desire is basically sinful but must somehow be dealt with (in the dark and taking as little time as possible). We may feel that we are far beyond the prudishness of the high Victorians who clothed piano legs in stockings so that they would not appear too suggestive. Yet shame is real, and it preys on all of us.

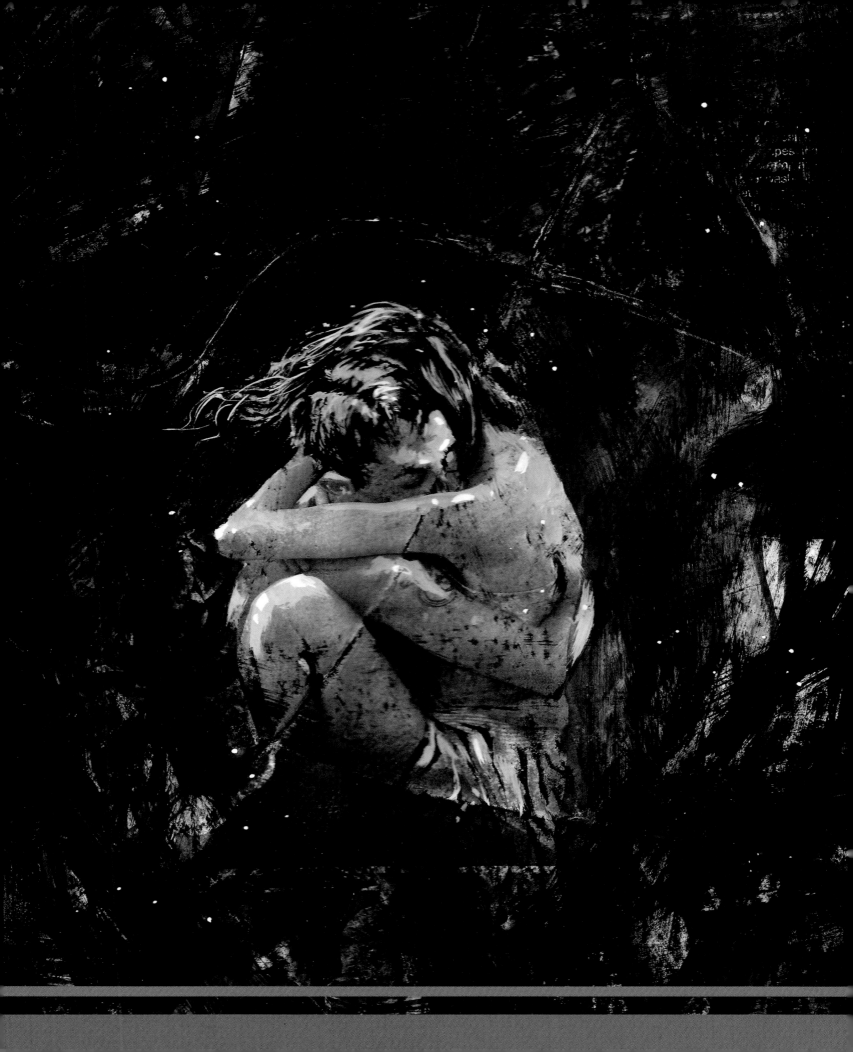

PLEASURE AND SHAME

The *Kama Sutra* can be read, first of all, as an antidote to shame. It celebrates carnality, making it a part of life to be seen in the clear light of day. The book is best known for its erotic illustrations, which depict the various positions for lovemaking. A few stretch the imagination almost as far as they stretch the lovers' bodies. The title is sometimes translated as 'Aphorisms on Love', but a better English version would be 'Instructions on Pleasure'. Sex is unadulterated pleasure when you enter the world of the *Kama Sutra*. The sexual organs are called 'the organs of pleasure'. As such they are not considered shameful, any more than the tongue is shameful because it brings the delights of eating or the skin is shameful because it brings the delights of touch.

A generation ago, when sexual liberation became a hot topic in the media, shame and repression were labeled, quite rightly, as enemies of happiness. But rarely were they seen as enemies of spirit, too. Sadly, the most religious people harbor the strongest prejudice against sex. It's no secret that 'purity', as religionists would have it, is a codeword for abstinence, and the purest spiritual life, as led by monks and nuns, is completely celibate. God, to put it bluntly, is not friendly to sex. Maybe he condoned it for a brief moment in the Garden of Eden, but once sex caught Satan's attention and became one of his chief weapons, a godly person has been expected to regard sex, not just with shame, but with a kind of righteous shame.

Shame makes you feel that you are not good enough and never can be. It's the last part that is so deadly to happiness. It makes millions of people agonize over their bodies for an entire lifetime. After all, if the body is regarded as shameful to begin with, not a day will go by that you won't be reminded of your sinful nature, your gross and indecent impulses, your ugliness that must be hidden behind clothes and make-up. (Children, although we sentimentally call them innocent, actually pick up feelings of shame at an extremely young age; as adults we can recall with a painful vividness the discovery that certain body parts and bodily functions are 'dirty'.)

The *Kama Sutra* couldn't be further from this view, which contains a blatant paradox: if God is an omniscient Creator, why would he create sex knowing that it would turn into an endless source of trouble? The pundit Vatsyayana, who wrote the *Kama Sutra*, is blessedly free of physical disgust, but he isn't naive. He understands lust; he depicts the stages of erotic obsession in great detail. For example, he gives the stages of romance: first, making eye contact, then exchanging longing glances, having erotic images come to mind that won't go away, followed by thinking of the beloved all the time, losing sleep, making excuses to meet, and finally culminating — if sexual contact is denied — with falling sick and dying.

The whole history of the romantic novel is written in those few observations. If you smile at the notion that sexual desire can make someone grow sick and die, you may be correct medically, but millions have wept over the death of Catherine Earnshaw pining for Heathcliff in *Wuthering Heights*, not to mention a thousand knights languishing for love in medieval romances and Shakespeare himself complaining of lovesickness in the sonnets — they all bear witness to the romantic view that we find in the *Kama Sutra*.

Vatsya knows what it feels like to covet your neighbor's wife: in fact, he gives detailed instructions on what to do in that situation. (Not that he condones it; in one place he forbids going through with the deed unless you have reached the stage of growing sick from desire and might die.) In many ways his audience was looking for common-sense sex advice, and we find that in abundance. For example, he gives 24 reasons why a married woman might turn down the advances of another man, such as:

- She still has affection for her husband
- She wants her children to be born in wedlock
- She lacks the right opportunity
- She feels offended by the man coming on too familiarly
- She thinks she is above or below the man socially
- She fears that he will run away
- She thinks he is too attached to his male friends
- She suspects that his intentions aren't serious
- She fears they will be discovered
- She just wants to remain friends

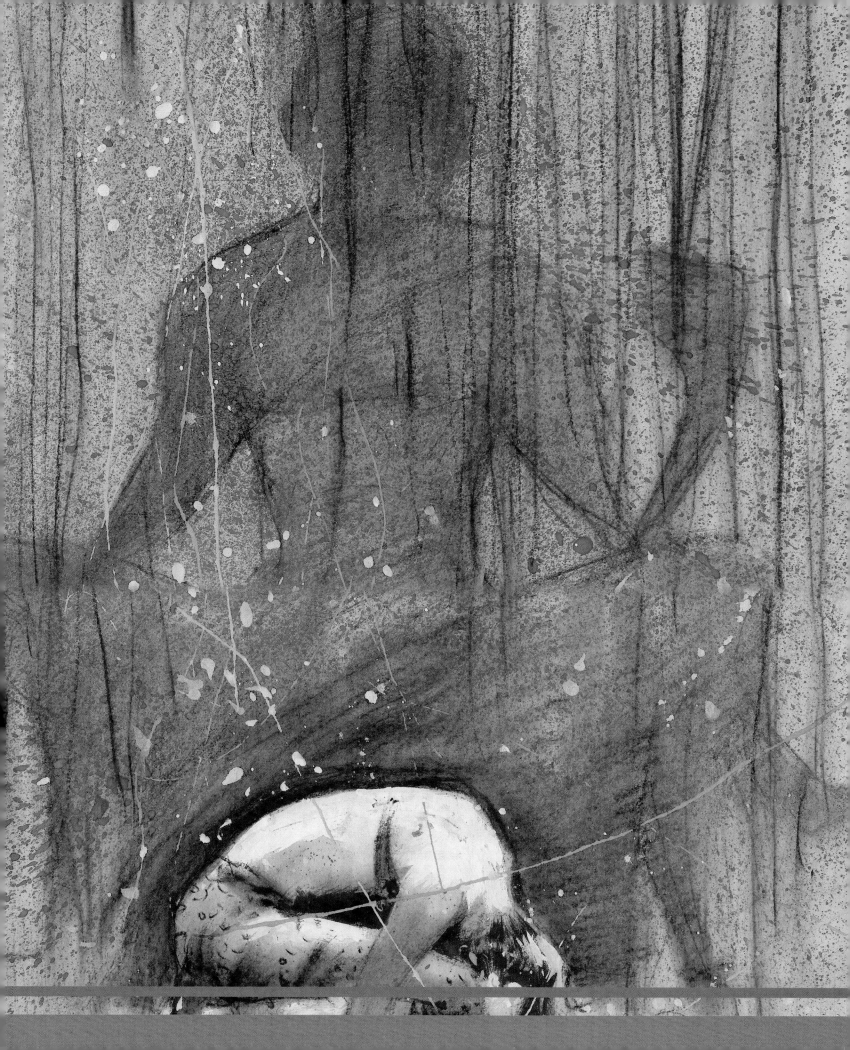

Fourteen more reasons to go, but already the reader senses that this is not a dusty old text; most of the time the *Kama Sutra* feels contemporary. Nor is this a lascivious *Penthouse* column on how to cheat — if anything, there are too many cautions laid out. The listing goes on to inform us that a married woman may say no because she is bashful, fears being discovered, despairs of not being perfect enough, or is put off by the possibility of being dominated. Amusingly, Vatsya remembers to mention that she may dislike the man's gray hair, scruffy appearance, or lack of worldly knowledge.

Yet for all his candid talk, Vatsya doesn't say that cheating is a sin, forbidden by God. He doesn't think that way, even though he lived as a monk. He tells us, in fact, that he wrote his book while in a state of 'deep contemplation of God'. But despite his frequent recourse to Holy Writ — meaning the accumulation of thousands of years of spiritual documents, many of which are now lost — Vatsya is refreshingly liberal, astonishingly so for his time. He has no qualms about premarital sex; he constantly advises men to pay attention to the desires of women. In fact, despite the social milieu which granted women no real equality, in the bedroom Vatsya insists that the playing field is even. Nor does he take a subtle route to misogyny by turning women into femmes fatales — to him, every desire is legitimate, no matter which gender has that desire, and all are equally entitled to find fulfillment. There is not a breath of social feminism in this book, in that men are seen to be the superior sex, but sexual feminism couldn't look to a better place to find its origins.

The *Kama Sutra* is actually erotic to read, despite its many practical sections. It keeps a sense of humor about sex, and when he wants to, Vatsyayana can whisk us off to the fantasy world of the *Arabian Nights*, as witness this passage, with its subtle witty ending:

> *Nowhere is as poorly guarded as a harem, and no women are more accessible than the wives of the king. An enterprising young man can choose any number of ways to get inside. Hidden in a barrel or masquerading as a maid, he can easily get past the lazy sentries and overworked servants. Another possibility is to take a potion that will make him invisible — but the outcome of this is uncertain.*

Here, then, is a humane alternative to the West's long-held suspicion that human sexuality is one of God's botched jobs.

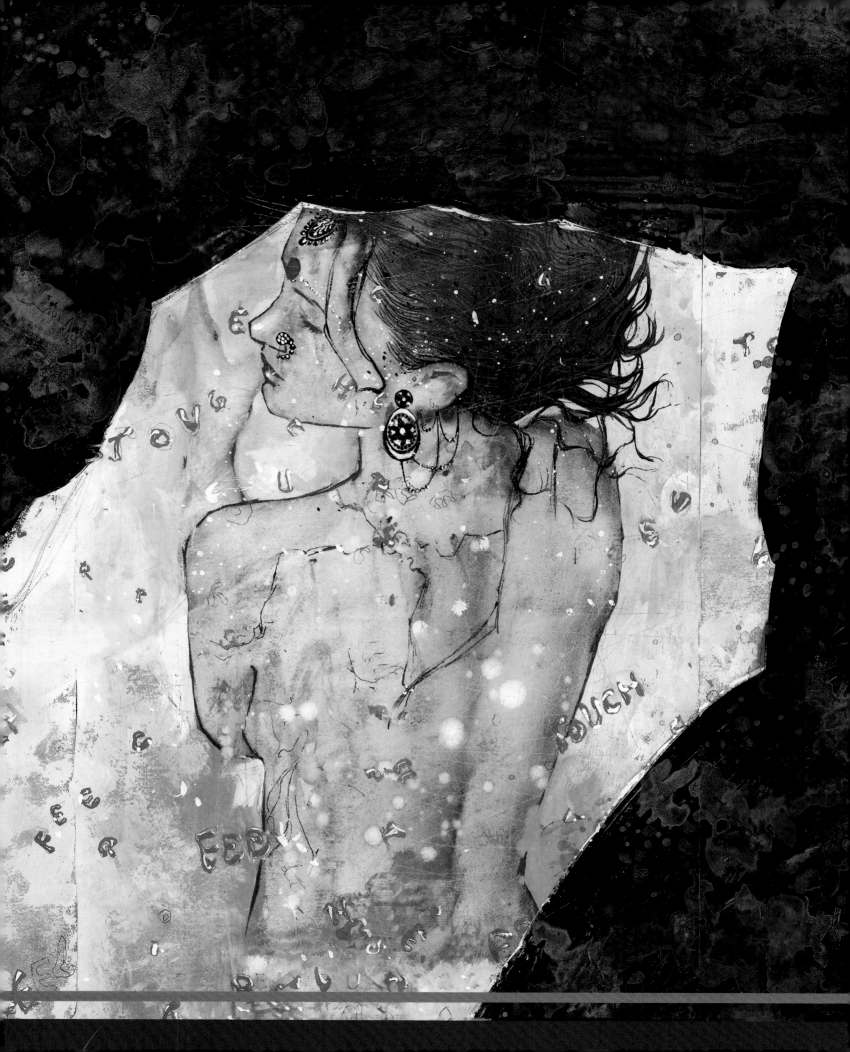

An Internal Shift

I decided to make my own English version of excerpts from the *Kama Sutra* because when anyone begins to actually read the text instead of just sneaking a peek at the pictures, one will find that an internal shift is beginning to take place. Shame and repression begin to stir from their hiding places. This works in different ways for different people. The ideal reader will be immensely relieved to run across a book that praises sex as a crucial aspect of the virtuous life — for the *Kama Sutra* is all about linking pleasure and virtue. It is not about being a slave to erotic desire, even though the prudes will insist that it is. Another reader may hope to find titillation here, only to discover a certain disgust creeping in. Should we really be reveling in our 'animal nature' this much? It's not in good taste, it's all, well, a bit seamy if not humiliating. While another reader may be outright shocked. 'You expect me to do that? To ask my wife (or husband) to go along?' Astonishingly intertwined bodies on a page are one thing; seeing yourself in the same situation is another.

This arousal of sexual feelings mixed with other, more negative, feelings is healthy. Self-discovery is only real when it acknowledges negative reactions and starts to purify them. So the second reason to call the *Kama Sutra* spiritual is that it encourages self-discovery. Until sex is part of your complete self — including your spiritual self — you do not truly understand who you are.

Thanks to the Internet, I've been asked tens of thousands of questions about spiritual life. Hundreds of questioners ask exactly what we all ponder about: What happens after we die? Do I have a soul? Who is God? People worry constantly about evil, getting sick, growing old. Perhaps the largest bulk of questions are about relationships and how to make one's family life more spiritual. Almost none, however, have been about sex. In a way this amazes me, because the truth about sex, and love in general, is that it remains the most powerful spiritual experience that most of us will have in our lifetimes. What is it like to be in love?

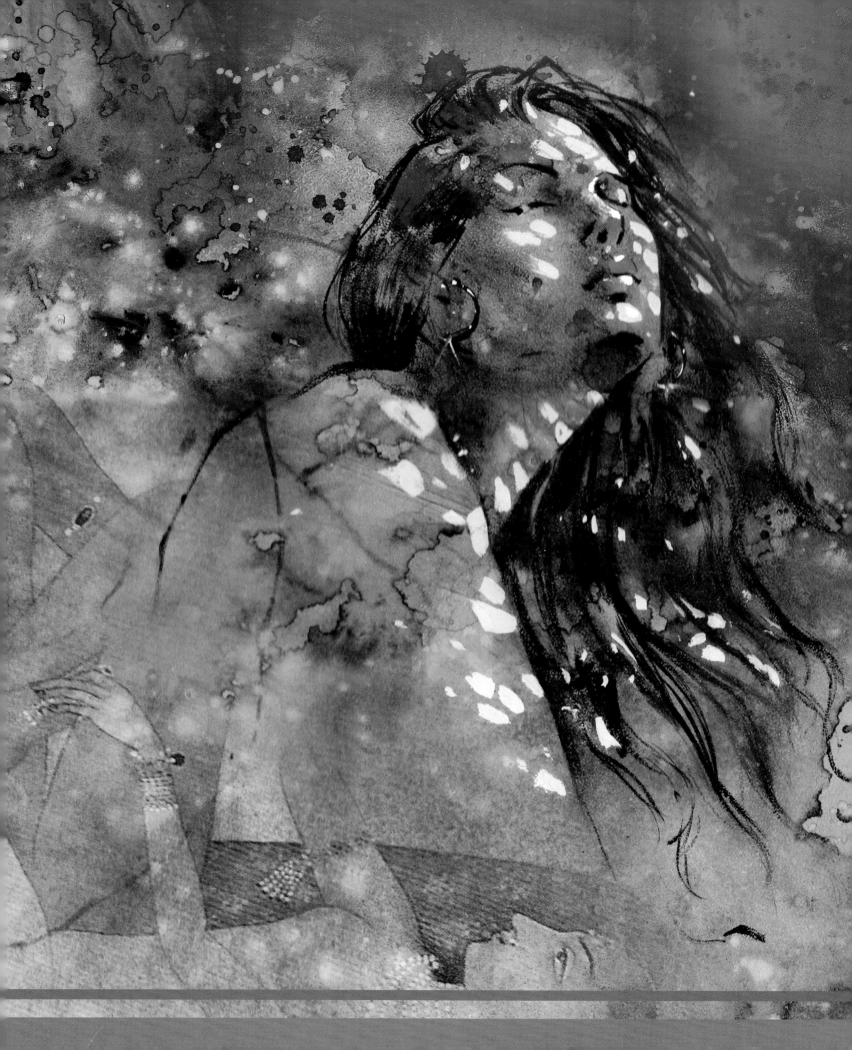

- You feel accepted and understood.

- You feel more complete, as if an invisible presence is filling you up.

- You imagine that you can do anything — life is suddenly open to all possibilities.

- You experience ecstasy in ordinary things: a glance, the touch of a hand, light falling on your beloved's face.

- Your self is expanded far beyond the petty limitations that were so confining before you fell in love.

I could catalog many more shifts in awareness that lovers experience, but they all have one thing in common. They exactly mirror the transcendent state of the greatest saints and sages. In spiritual terms you are not deluding yourself when you fall in love. You are seeing yourself as you truly are. Unfortunately, the spiritual exaltation of love is usually temporary. Once you fall out of love, there is a thumping return to earth. Love is no longer an amazing, transformative gift. It becomes something else, far more ordinary. Or rather, we turn back into whatever we were before love changed us.

One could take two views of this all-too-brief interlude. Either falling in love was a kind of vacation into pleasant madness, a brief respite to be enjoyed as long as it lasted (while others look on smiling patiently) before real life intrudes with all its harsh and mundane banality. Or you can look at falling in love as what real life is supposed to be. The first perspective follows Freud's 'reality principle', which demands that a psychologically healthy person harbor no idealistic illusions, no faith in a world beyond, no trust in the fickle impulses of subjectivity. This sounds so sensible that few people dare to take the second perspective, which recognizes a higher reality, compared to which the material world is the illusion, a multicolored Maya that fools the senses for ever and ever.

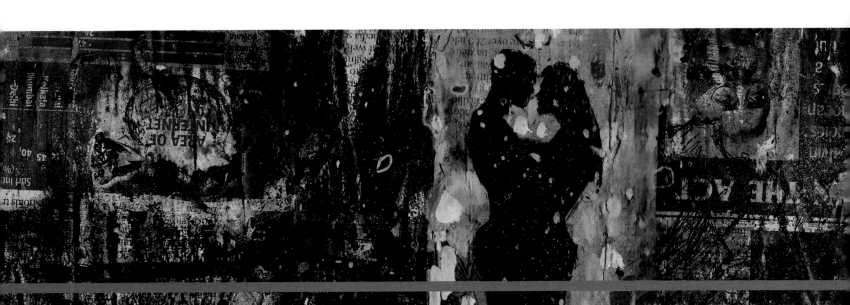

The *Kama Sutra* is a perfect litmus test for which view you really trust. If you are a realist, then the book is merely a sex manual, to be used the way a gourmet uses a cookbook of subtle, refined recipes. If you are spiritual, the book is a door to peak experiences and you approach its instructions the way a priest would approach a religious ritual. Most of us are stark realists. Sex is not among our peak experiences. By this I don't simply mean a peak of pleasure. A good sex life gives rise to much pleasure; it brings you into intimate connection with someone you love, whose body you crave to touch. But true peak experiences contain much more than this: they are glimpses into the reality of the soul. Look back at the list of changes that happen when a person falls in love. The feelings of completeness and power, of all possibilities being laid out before one, of a world where everyday details shimmer in ecstasy — these are the very qualities of the soul.

Modern India is praised for at long last starting to catch up with the technologies of the West, and it has become commonplace to hear an Indian accent on the other end of the line when we call about our credit-card bill. Yet in some ways the old India far outstripped the new, only to be ignored in those areas where the greatest value lies. (One must remember that today's India is a country where the movie censors forbid onscreen kissing, and where an actress creates a front-page scandal if she leaves the country and happens to kiss a man in a foreign film.) Old India had a vision of life, one so complete that no activity was divorced from it, including sex.

The one aspect of the *Kama Sutra* that might baffle and bore many readers is its relentless thoroughness. Why so many, many sexual positions? Why such endless detail about a carnal act that for most people occupies less than half an hour about three times a month (an average statistic in the United States)? The answer is that the spiritual tradition of India had to be this thorough because it saw life as something to be completely understood and mastered.

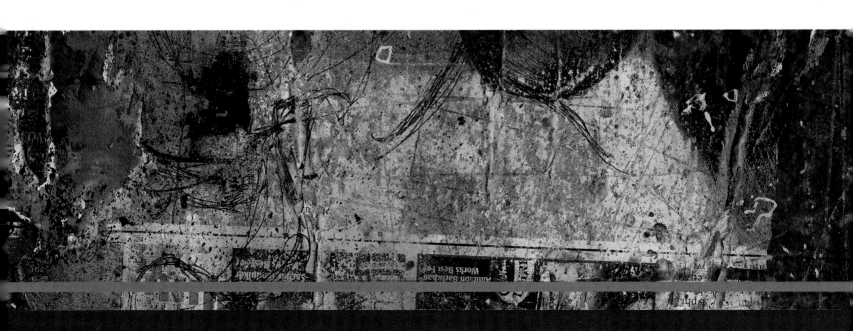

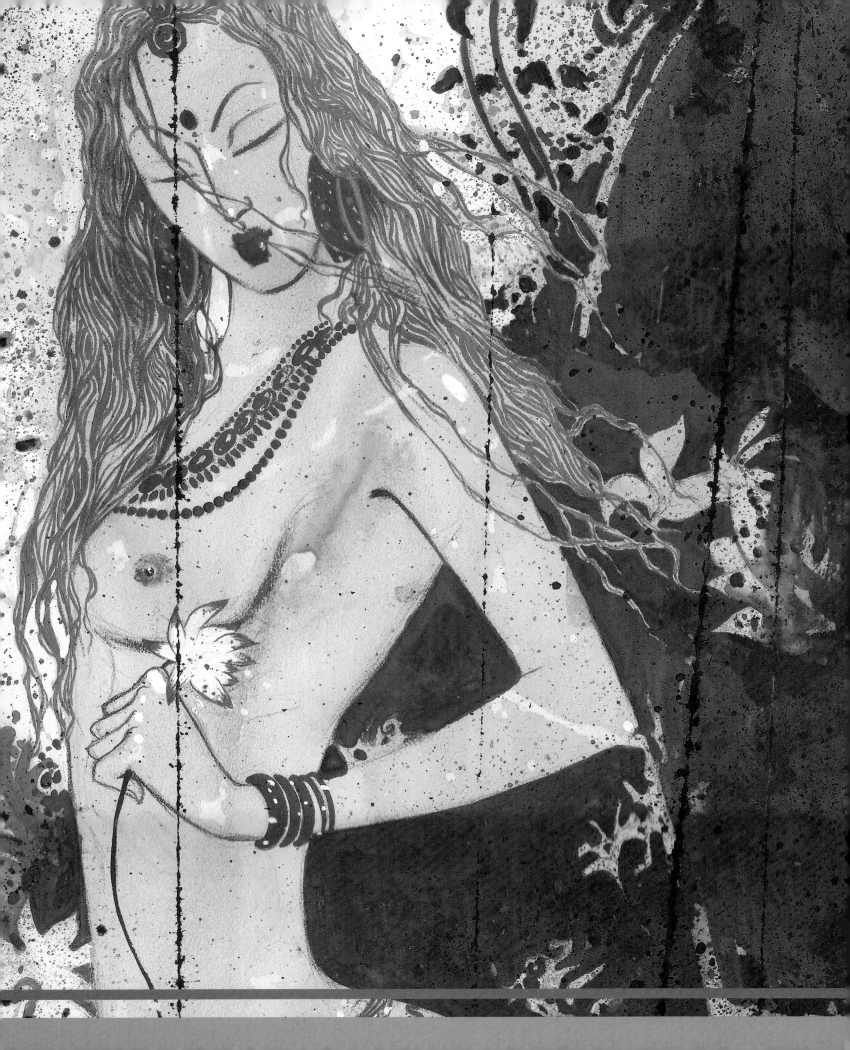

THE FOUR GOALS OF LIFE

Every Indian child for the past three thousand years has grown up being guided by four main goals in life. They are:

- Desire, pleasure through the five senses (Kama)
- Success, including wealth, friends, and possessions (Artha)
- Virtue, adherence to universal law (Dharma)
- Liberation of the self (Moksha)

Originally these were the names of gods; they are still considered divine attributes. Which means they were not invented by a particular culture but rather came down to us as the innate value of life itself. In its opening pages the *Kama Sutra* raises possible objections to learning about sex. One is that desire, being physical and present all the time, doesn't require expert advice; it should just be taken naturally. (Shades of parents in the era before sex education, who hoped that their teenagers would learn about sex on their own, without 'the talk'.) The answer to this objection is that 'brute nature' is different from human nature. Animals in the wild mate randomly, the females are in heat only for specific months of the year, and the act of intercourse is crude and swift. Among humans, however, sex is a refined pleasure and should be treated as seriously as growing rich or being virtuous. Lovemaking, one of the most basic outlets of Kama, is both an art and a science.

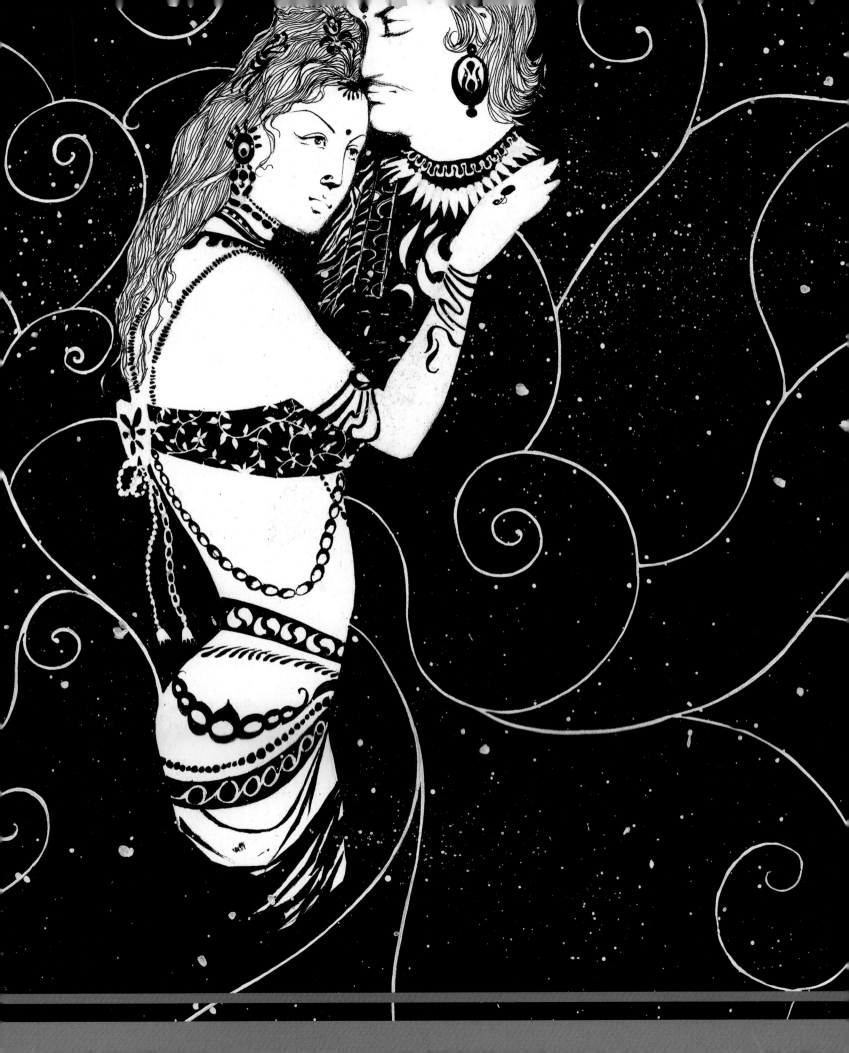

In the larger scheme the four goals of life are connected to one another, and they cascade in reverse order.

- **Moksha** or liberation comes first; it is the primary goal toward which everything else aims
- **Dharma** or virtuous living is needed for the proper orientation toward achieving freedom
- **Artha** or material success is good on its own terms, but it must serve the agenda of the soul; otherwise money and possessions are just as binding as wrong actions
- On the lowest rung **Kama** or desire is also good on its own terms, but lacking a spiritual component it vanishes without a trace

With this hierarchy in mind, modern society has managed to turn the four goals of life upside down. For what do people live for primarily but to fulfill their every desire, to be materially successful, and to enjoy respectable social standing? Last, and often very least, comes spirituality, which is usually confined to irregular attendance at church or temple. The soul's freedom, or Moksha, is dreamed of as a reward in heaven after we die. Even though sensual desire is the lowest goal of life, the *Kama Sutra* emphasizes, over and over, that all four must be 'practiced in harmony, never clashing with one another'. Sensuality is not glorified in its own right; it attains its glory as an aspect of a spiritual journey.

If you treat the *Kama Sutra* like a sex manual it will certainly serve the modern topsy-turvy approach to life, and like pleasure itself will vanish as a once-intriguing, now-forgotten experience. Another temptation in a long line of temptations. To read the book as it was intended, we have to overturn our hierarchy of personal values, putting liberation on top instead of at the bottom. And to do that, one has to read the actual book itself, which I have excerpted in the following section.

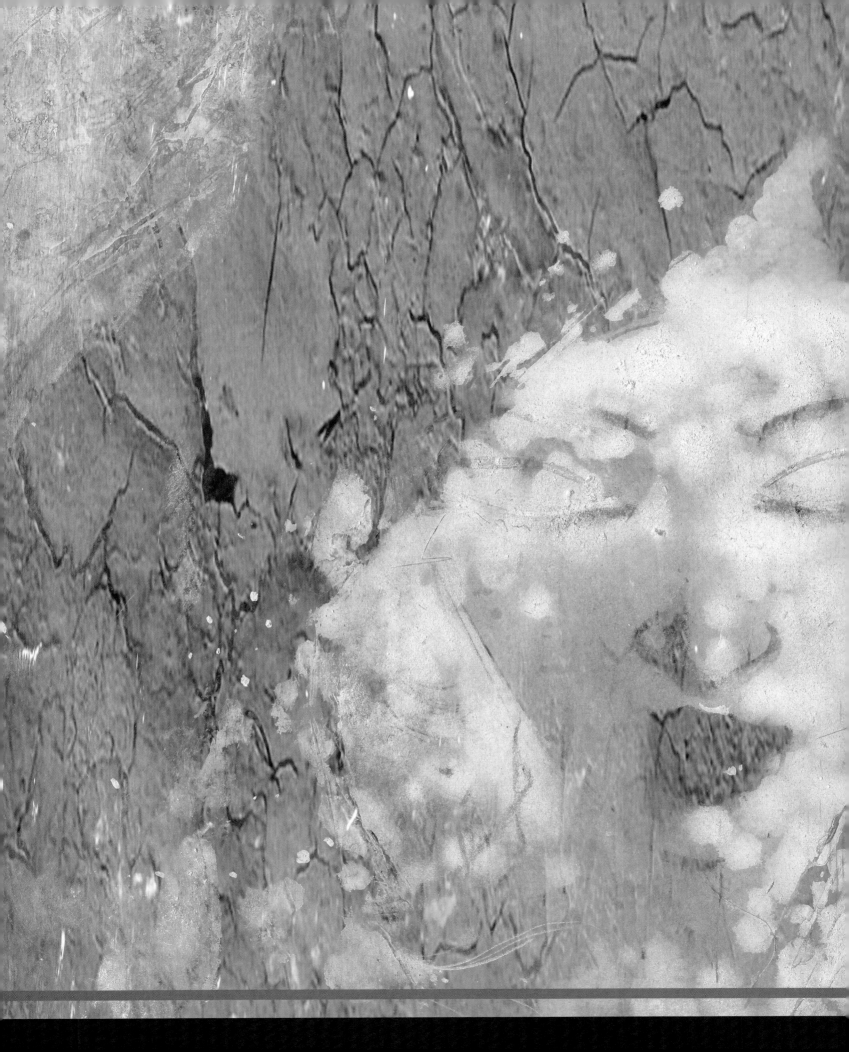

CHAPTER 2

READING THE KAMA SUTRA

*T*here follow key passages from the **Kama Sutra** that give the full flavor of the book. This isn't a book that keeps to one tone. Any given paragraph can be wise, cynical, ribald, witty, fantastic, irreverent, manipulative, and clinical by turns.

The only tone it avoids is the smirking and lascivious. There is even room for Machiavellian behavior (I am thinking of one passage where Vatsyayana declares that a man can seduce a married woman without sin if he has an ulterior motive, such as wanting to murder her husband!) If one aspect of a spiritual text is its ability to break through our boundaries and shock us into new perceptions, the Kama Sutra eminently qualifies, despite the fact that so much is about flesh instead of spirit. No matter how unpredictable or even bizarre it becomes, one thing remains constant: a refusal to be ashamed of sexual pleasure.

On every erotic topic Vatsyayana tries to sound as worldly and assured as he can, a weakness that almost all sex manuals, then and now, fall into. He can be intolerably cruel in his worldliness, as when he lists those women who are easy to seduce and includes hunchbacks, dwarves, widows, and mothers who have lost a child. Of course, there is also a fund of sound sexual advice about pleasing one another that lovers continue to benefit from.

Many readers will be surprised to learn that the famous sections on sexual positions form only part of a single chapter. I have restricted myself to scattered excerpts taken from every part of the *Kama Sutra* because a great deal of the book is by now a curious relic — like all books, it was a product of its times. Vatsya assumes that his reader belongs to one of the four traditional castes of India. He believes that sexual partners should be paired off as equals, by which he means that they belong to the same caste and the same physical type (hence his discussion of elephant men, rabbit men, deer women, etc., which I have skipped over). He takes polygamy for granted, also that men are more sexually impetuous than women and naturally take the lead as pursuers and seducers. Even so, after all the quaintness and historical dust have been cleared away, there is much left that is still fascinating and revealing about human nature.

The book is full of customs peculiar to northern India somewhere between the first and sixth century AD but Vatsya assures us that he has distilled many ancient texts, now lost, amounting to hundreds of books. He sometimes quotes verses from these other authorities. No one really knows who Vatsya was or when he lived; it is assumed, because he tells us so, that he worked from even more ancient Sanskrit texts on lovemaking. All that is certain is that his *Kama Sutra* is the oldest surviving Indian writing on the art of love. The earliest English translation was made by Sir Richard Burton in 1883; like almost everyone else who has followed, I've relied on it when making my own version. Burton's approach to sex was chivalrous. Some of his flowery style is worth preserving, and at times I have felt free to phrase in a poetic way. But where Vatsyayana is frank and candid, I have tried to be that way, too.

THE KAMA SUTRA OF VATSYAYANA

PLEASURE AND THE GOALS OF LIFE

Human beings, whose lifetime is allotted at one hundred years, should pursue three goals in life: virtue (Dharma), material success (Artha) and desire or pleasure (Kama) each in its own way and its own time, but in harmony so that they do not clash with one another. Childhood should be devoted to religious education; youth and middle age to Artha and Kama; old age to Dharma. In this way one seeks to gain final liberation, or Moksha, to end the cycle of birth and rebirth.

Kama includes all enjoyment derived from the five senses, assisted by the mind and the soul. The common factor is that a particular sense comes into contact with an object of desire, and when contact is made, being conscious of the pleasure this creates is Kama.

Kama is to be learned from the *Kama Sutra* — the text devoted to pleasure — and from life experience.

When all three goals of life come together, virtue has priority over material success, and material success has priority over pleasure. Courtesans and public women (prostitutes), because of their profession, place pleasure first, but these are exceptions to the general rule.

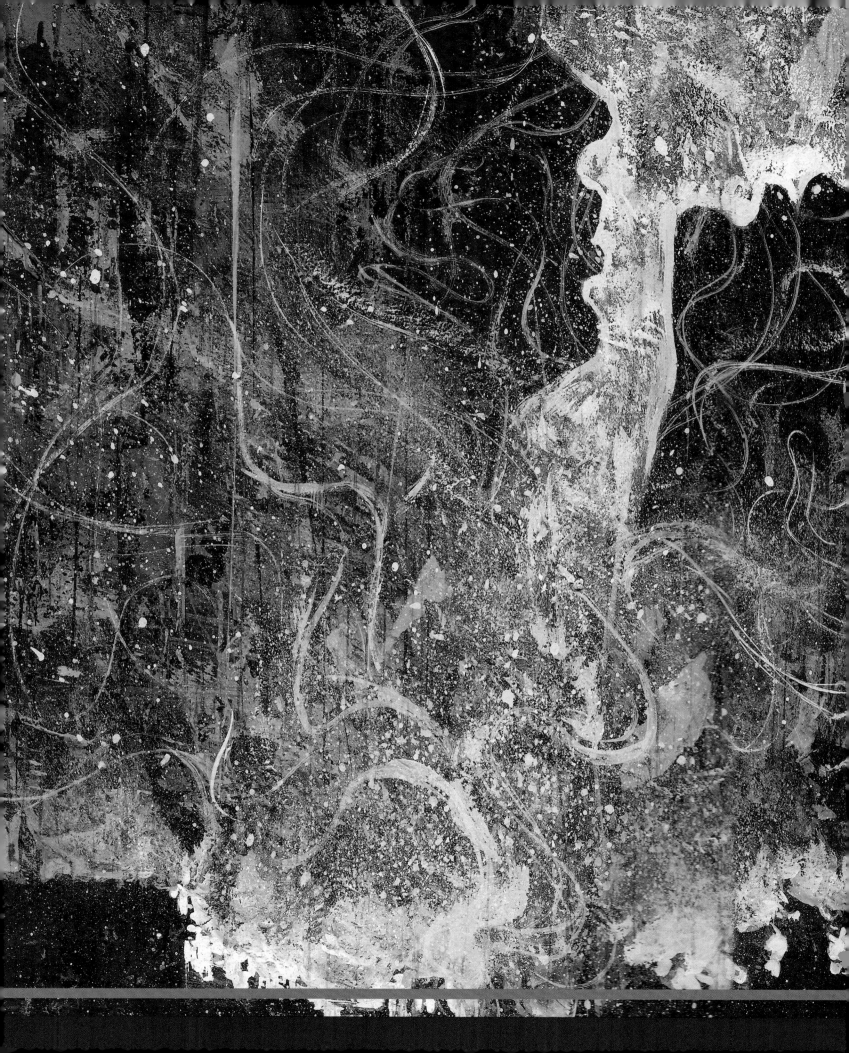

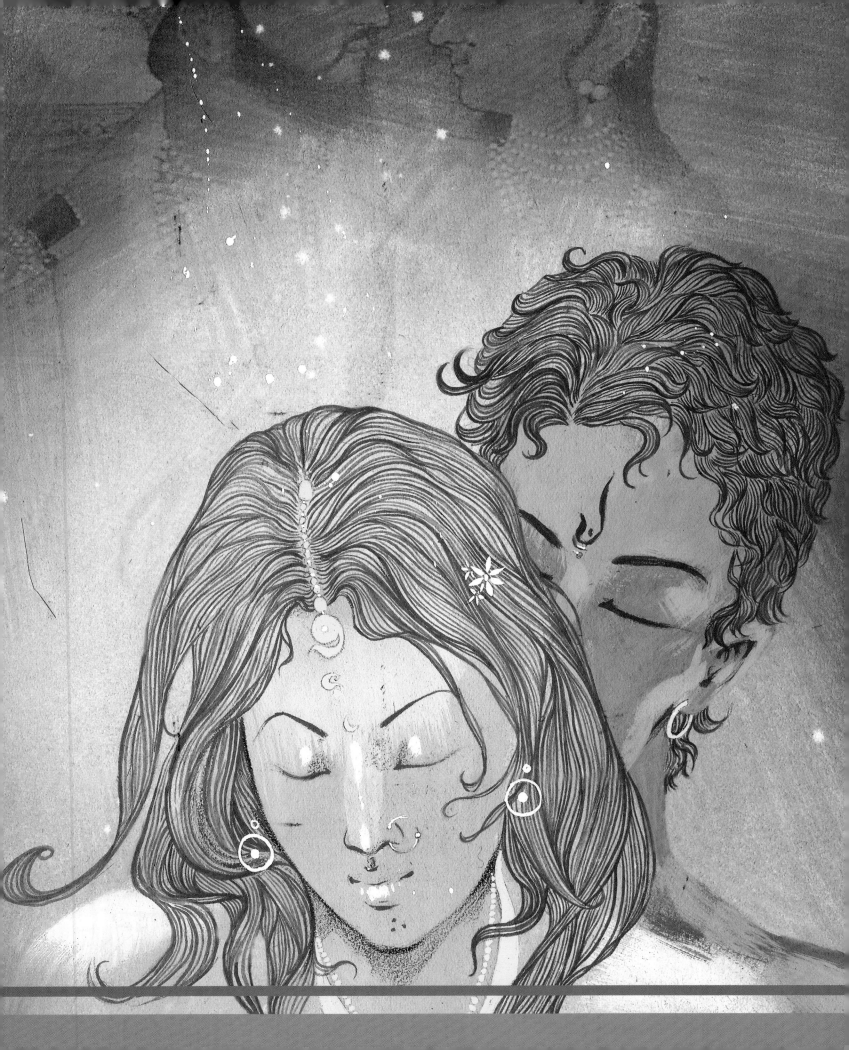

Objection: Some authorities declare that Dharma and Artha can be learned from books, the first because religious matters are abstract and do not belong to this world, the second because material success depends upon learning specific skills. But pleasure, they say, doesn't need to be studied. We see animals practicing sexual behavior, which is found naturally everywhere in creation.

Reply: The comparison isn't valid. Men and women need the *Kama Sutra* to learn the proper means to pursue pleasure correctly. Among animals the situation is different because their behavior is unrestrained; the females are in heat only for a certain time and no other; and their intercourse is not preceded by any thought.

Objection: Others object that pleasure should not be sought after because it interferes with the superior goals of virtue and material success. Sexual pleasure is looked down on by people of merit. Sex brings a man into distress; it puts him in contact with persons of low degree, who lead him into unrighteous behavior and all kinds of impurity. They make him forget the future; they tempt him to become lazy and disorderly. Finally, they cause him to lose his credibility, to be unwelcome in respectable houses and despised by everyone, including himself. Notoriously, men who solely give themselves over to pleasure wind up ruining themselves and their families.

Reply: This is an untenable objection given that pleasure is as necessary to the body and to one's sense of wellbeing as food. Moreover, there are pleasures that directly result from virtue and success. One should pursue pleasure in moderation and with caution. No one refrains from cooking just because beggars might try to get the food once it's made, or from sowing seed because deer might eat the crops once they're grown. As for fear of the life to come, the three goals of life should be pursued without fear of their future effects. If all three, or even two, or even one of them are in harmony and support the others, there is no danger. But if any action harms the pursuit of the other goals, it shouldn't be performed.

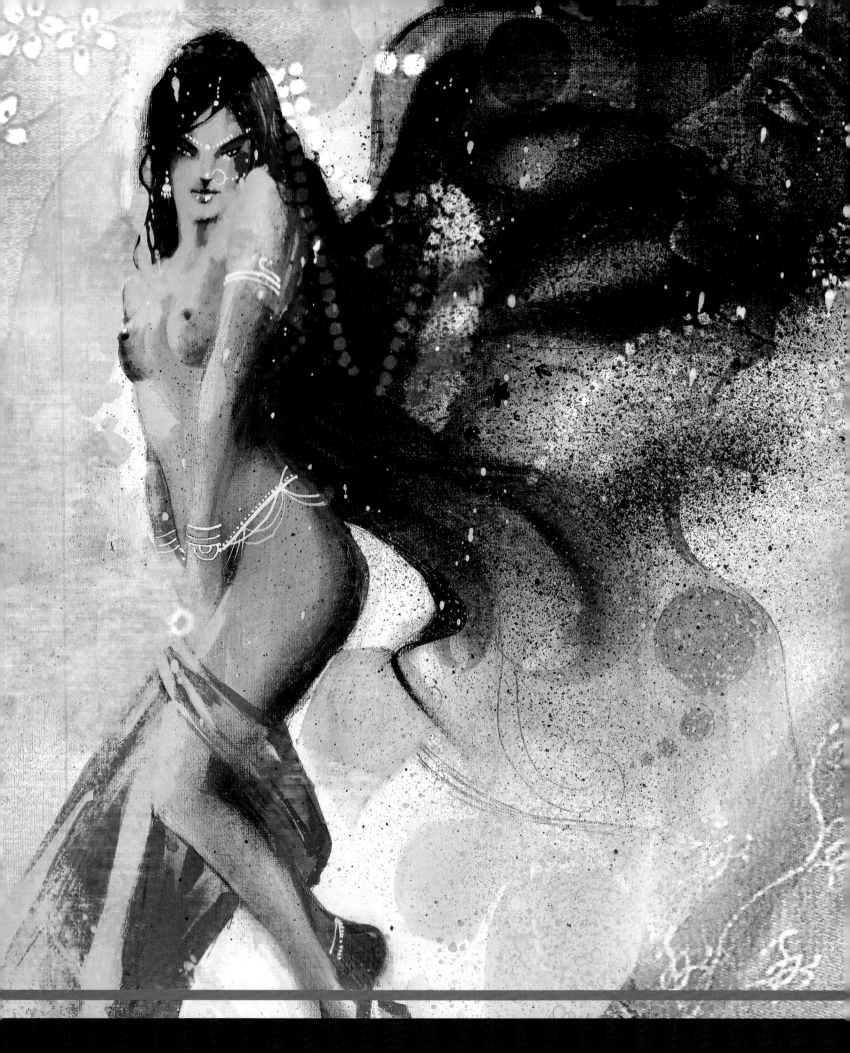

ENJOYING WOMEN (WITHOUT SIN)

There are three kinds of women who fall under the category of Nayika, a woman with whom a man can enjoy sexual pleasure without sin: virgins, women who have been married twice, and courtesans or public women. (Only the first is suitable for marrying and bearing children; the other two are for pleasure alone.) But there is a fourth kind of Nayika, a married woman who is resorted to for a specific purpose, and this purpose is not for progeny or pleasure. Instead, a man may be following some ulterior motive, such as:

- This woman is independent and self-willed. Other men have enjoyed her before me. Therefore, even if she is of a higher caste than mine, I can sleep with her without violating the laws of Dharma (the religious duties for each caste).

- This woman has won the heart of a powerful man, her husband, and has mastery over him. Her husband happens to be the friend of my enemy; therefore, if I manage to win the wife over, she will persuade him to abandon my enemy.

- This woman can get her powerful husband to favor me, while at present he is turned against me and does me harm.

- This woman is in a position to advance a friend of mine or ruin one of my enemies, or otherwise aid me in accomplishing something difficult.

- By winning this woman over, I can kill her husband, whose riches I covet.

- I am poor and unable to support myself, but if I unite myself with this woman, I can have her money risk free. I really need the money, and this is a way to get some without difficulty.

- This woman is madly in love with me and knows all my weaknesses. If I don't sleep with her, she will tell everyone what they are, and then my reputation will be ruined. Or she could ruin me by bringing a false accusation that would be hard to disprove. Or she might turn her powerful husband against me, since she has influence over him, or even might join my enemies herself.

- This woman's husband has violated my wives; therefore, I will seduce his in return.

- This woman is sheltering an enemy of the king's. I've been ordered to kill him, and I can only get at him by sleeping with her.

- I love another woman, who is this woman's best friend. If I sleep with this woman, I can get to the one I really want.

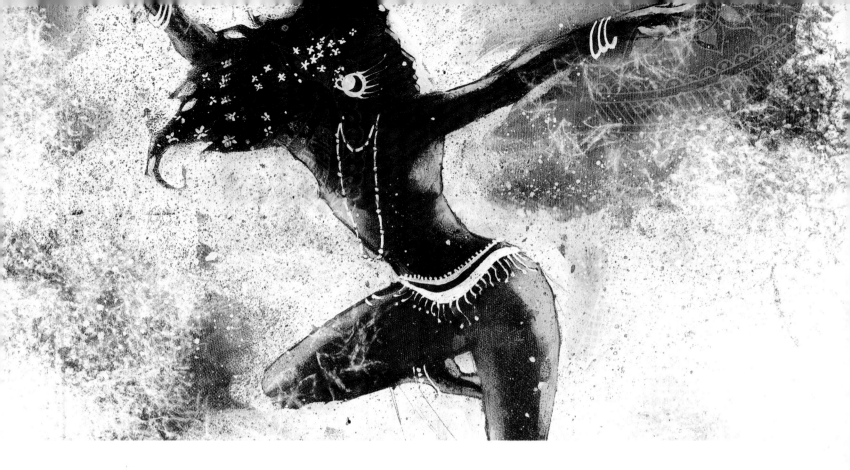

For these and similar other reasons, a man may sleep with another man's wife. But it needs to be strictly understood that there have to be special reasons; it is not for carnal desire.

The following women are not to be enjoyed at all:

- Lepers
- Lunatics
- Women of no caste
- Women who tell secrets
- Women who ask for sex in public
- Women who are too pale and white
- Women who are too dark and black
- Women who smell bad
- Near relations
- A female friend
- Someone leading the life of an ascetic or nun
- Finally, any wives of a friend, relative, learned Brahmin, or the king

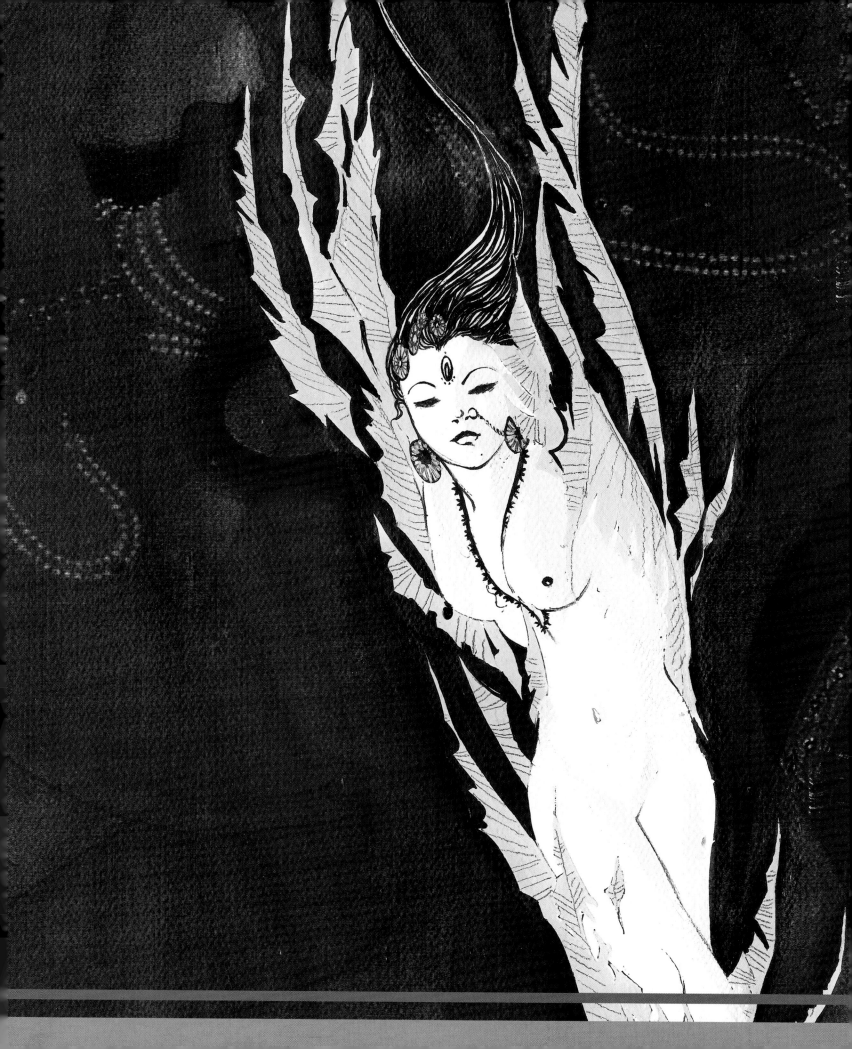

MALE AND FEMALE PASSION

Men of small passion are called that because their desire while having sex is not very great, their semen is scanty, and they can't bear the embrace of a passionate woman. Men of middling passion have more desire than this, and then there are men who are full of passion. Likewise, women are said to have the same three degrees of passion. There are also three categories for how much time the sex act takes. Some men take a short time, others a middling or long time. All this (along with the size of a man's penis and the depth of a woman's vagina) determines suitable ways of having sex between different kinds of men and women. From the various combinations of these factors, there are innumerable ways to perform the sex act. Each person derives pleasure in his or her own way, irrespective of the workings (sexual characteristics) of the other.

However, on this point there's a disagreement concerning women. The sage Auddalika says, 'Women do not have a man's emission. Men simply discharge their desire, while women, from their awareness of desire, feel a certain kind of satisfaction that they can't describe. The evidence of this is that men are satisfied as soon as they discharge while women are not.' The objection to this opinion is on the grounds that if a man is the type who takes a long time, the woman loves him more, while if he takes only a short time, she will be dissatisfied with him. This circumstance proves, according to some, that the woman also has an emission (i.e. orgasm).

But this opinion about how women gain pleasure overlooks that it can take a long time to satisfy a woman (to the point of orgasm), and during that time she is also having great pleasure. It's only natural that she would want this to continue. A verse applies here: 'By union with a man, the lust or desire of a woman is satisfied, and the consciousness of being pleasured is how she gains satisfaction.' At the outset of intercourse a woman's passion is middling, however, and she cannot bear the vigorous thrusting of her lover. Her passion increases by degrees until she ceases to think about her body, and finally she comes to the point where she wants intercourse to end.

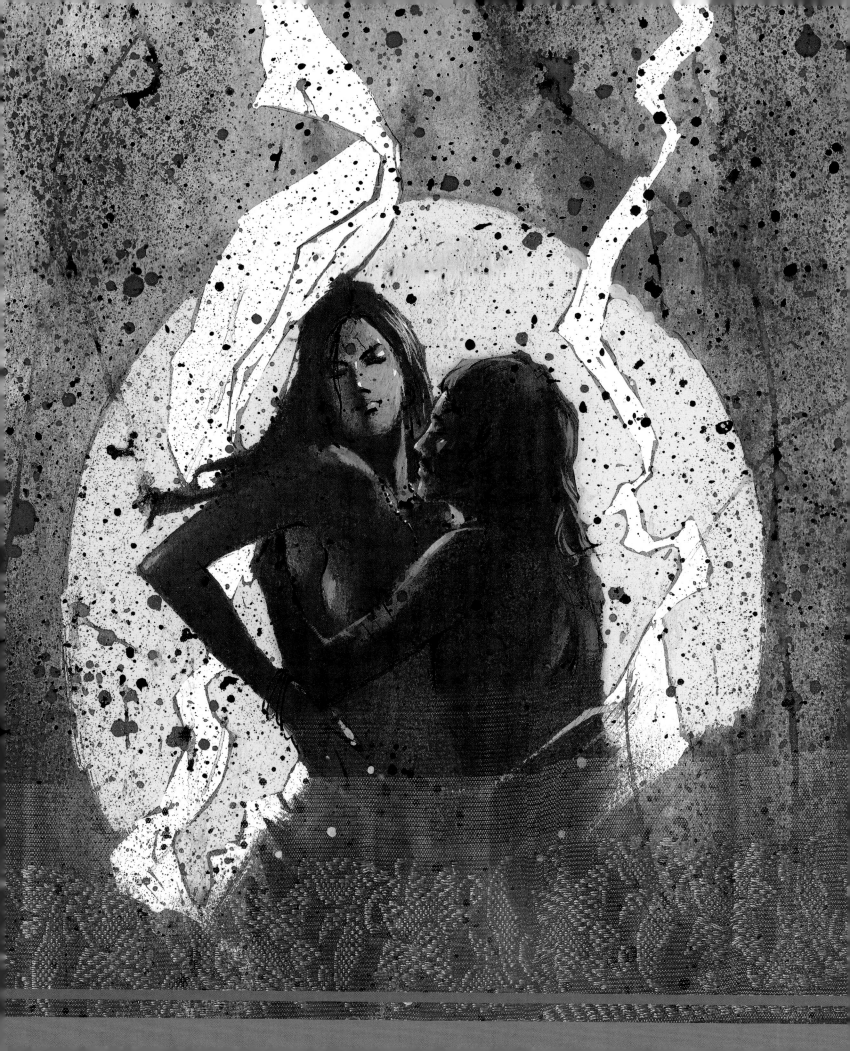

Objection: If men and women are of the same kind, engaged in bringing about the same result (orgasm), why should they go about it in such different ways? Shouldn't they work the same way?

Reply: The ways of working are different, and the consciousness of pleasure isn't the same in men and women. Men approach sex as the actor, women as the one acted upon. This doesn't operate sometimes one way, sometimes the other. From this way of working, a man's awareness of being united with a woman is not the same as a woman's awareness of being united with a man.

Yet someone might still object, if there is this difference in the ways of working, why don't men and women experience a different kind of pleasure from each other? This conclusion is groundless. It may be necessary for men and women to have different roles during sex, but they are seeking the same kind of pleasure from the act. When two rams butt heads, they both receive a shock at the same time. But men and women are configured differently, so even though they are performing the same act, they arrive at equal pleasure through two modes of working.

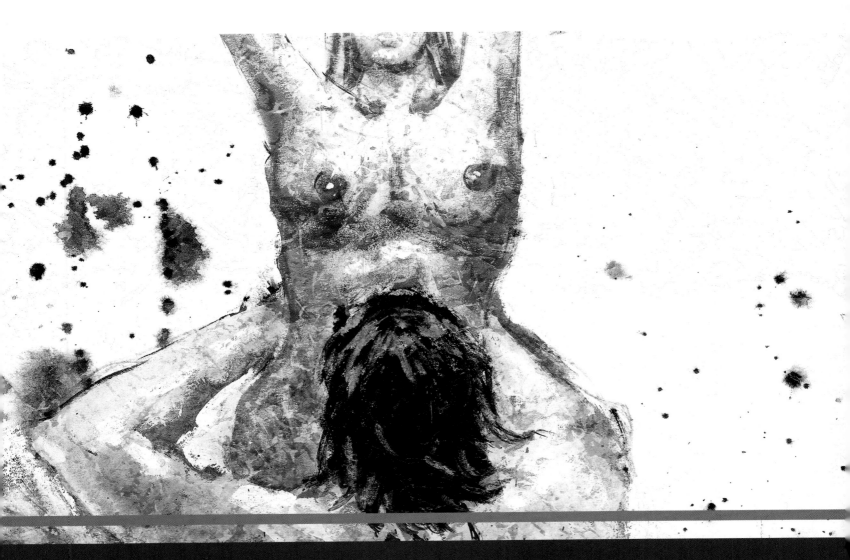

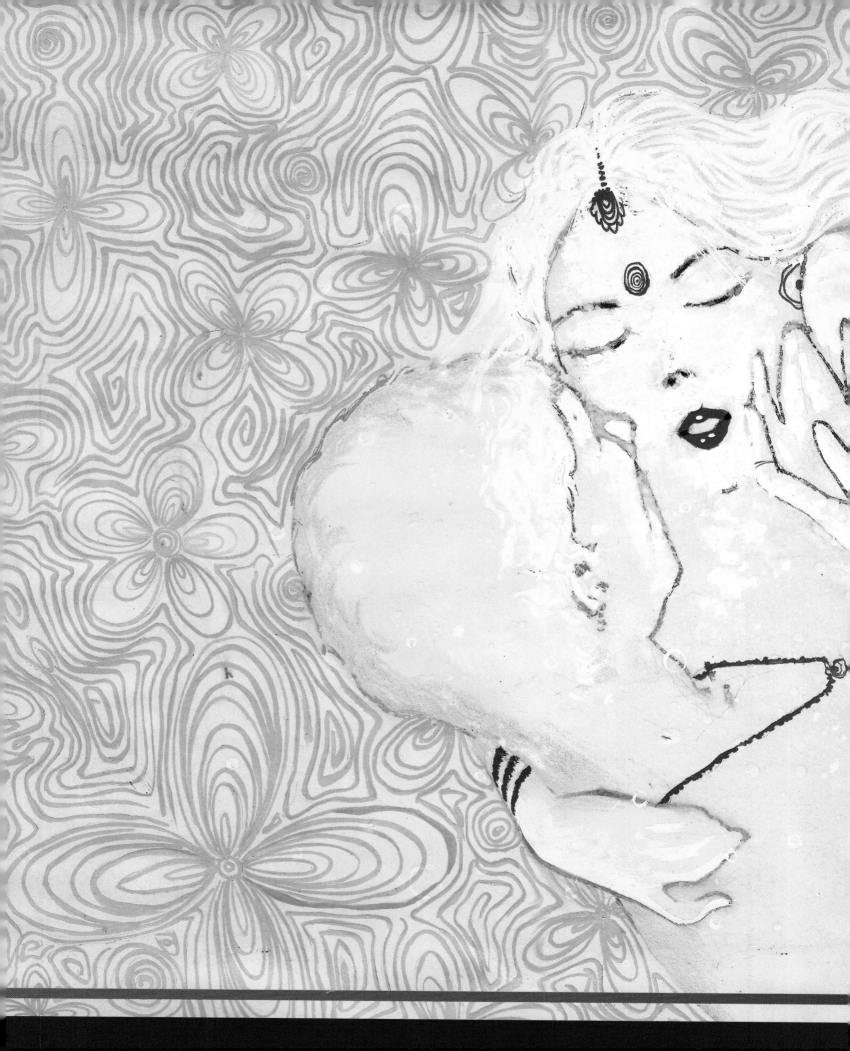

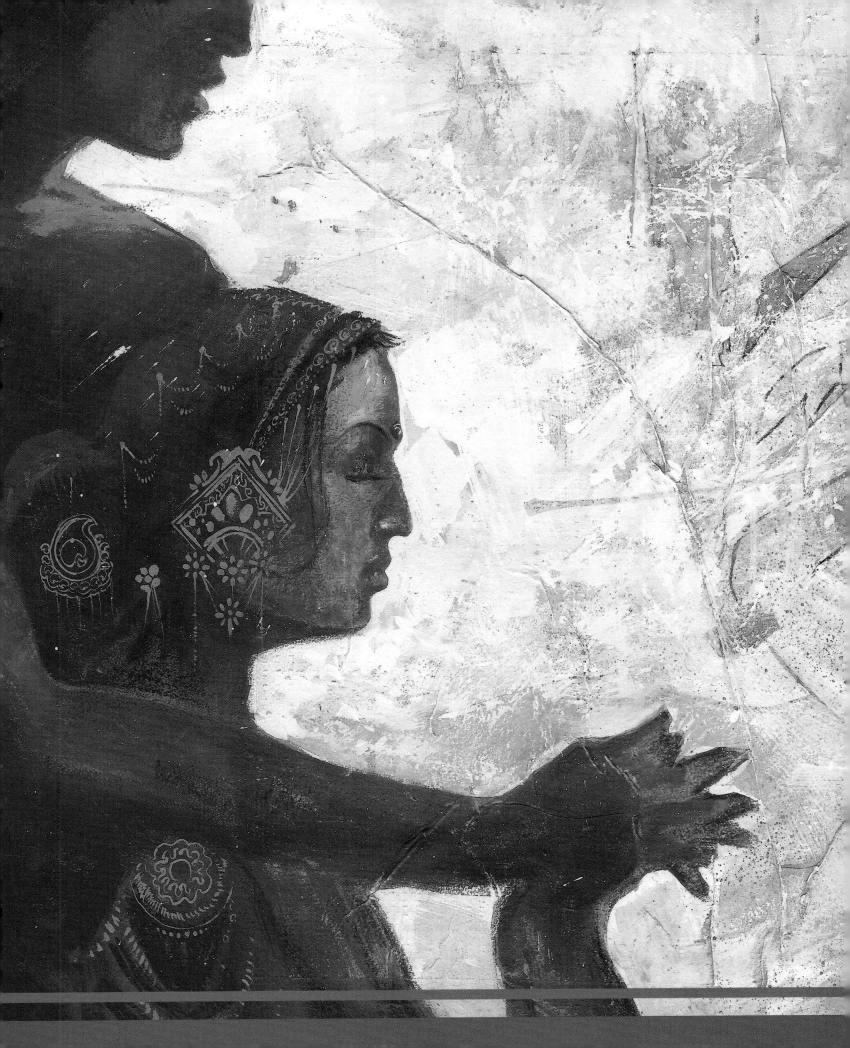

CATALOG OF EMBRACES

If a man happens to brush up against a woman, using some excuse or other, and touches her either on the front or the side, this is called 'the touching embrace'.

A woman is alone with a man someplace and bends over, as if picking up something from the ground. If her breasts touch him and he fondles them, that is called 'the piercing embrace'. These two embraces occur between two people who aren't yet speaking freely to each other about sex.

If two lovers are out strolling, say at night or out in public, and their bodies rub up against each other, this is called 'a rubbing embrace'. When this contact leads to eagerly pushing one of them up against a wall or pillar, this is called 'a pressing embrace'. These two embraces belong to those who know exactly what their intentions are. As they continue, four kinds of embrace may arise: twining with each other like a creeper, like climbing a tree, like sesame seeds mixed with rice, or like water in milk.

In detail, if a woman clings to a man as closely as a vine to a tree, bends his face down to hers, and looks lovingly into his eyes with the desire to be kissed, that is 'the embrace of the creeper'. If she places one foot on the man's foot and the other on his thigh, one arm around his back and the other around his neck, sighing and cooing, this is 'climbing a tree', because it's as if she wants to climb up him so that she may be kissed. Both of these embraces take place while the lovers are standing.

When they lie down and embrace each other closely, in a tangle of arms and legs, rubbing their thighs together, they are 'mixing sesame seeds and rice'. If a couple is so in love that they cannot even think of pain or discomfort, their bodies squeeze so close that they could be melting into each other. This embrace, which can also be done with the woman sitting in the man's lap or standing up as well as in bed, is like 'mixing water and milk'. Both of these embraces occur during sexual intercourse.

Besides these eight embraces, one also finds lovers fondling a particular part of the body, such as embrace of the thighs, breasts, forehead, or the lower half of the woman's body from the navel down (Jaghana). Some authorities say that giving a shampoo is a kind of embrace, since two bodies come into contact, but Vatsya replies that washing the hair is done at different times and for a different purpose than love and therefore shouldn't be included among the embraces.

Lastly, there is a verse which says that when a man learns about these embraces, asks questions about them, or even overhears what they are, he immediately desires to enjoy them. Kinds of touching that aren't mentioned in the texts on love should be practiced at the time of intercourse if they increase passion and delight. The set-down rules of how to embrace a woman aid a man of middling sexual drive, but when the wheel of love is madly turning, rules and order go out the window!

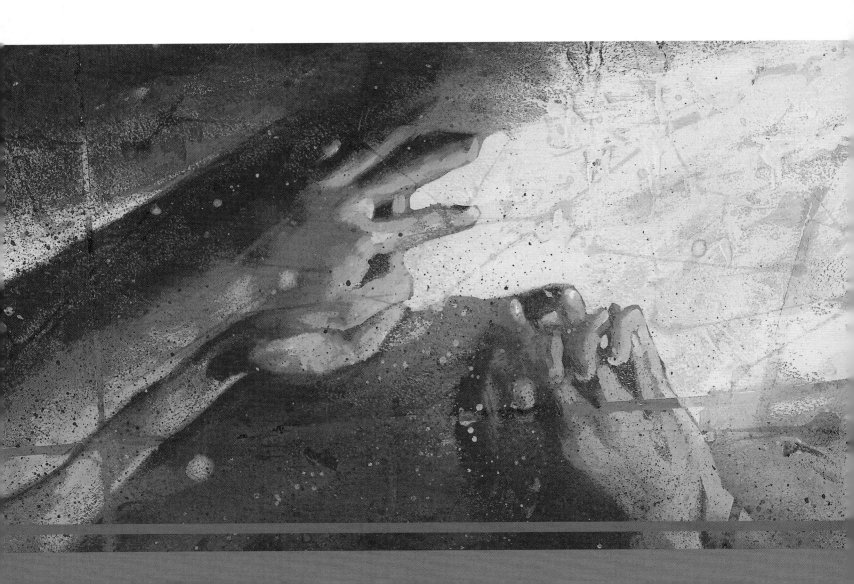

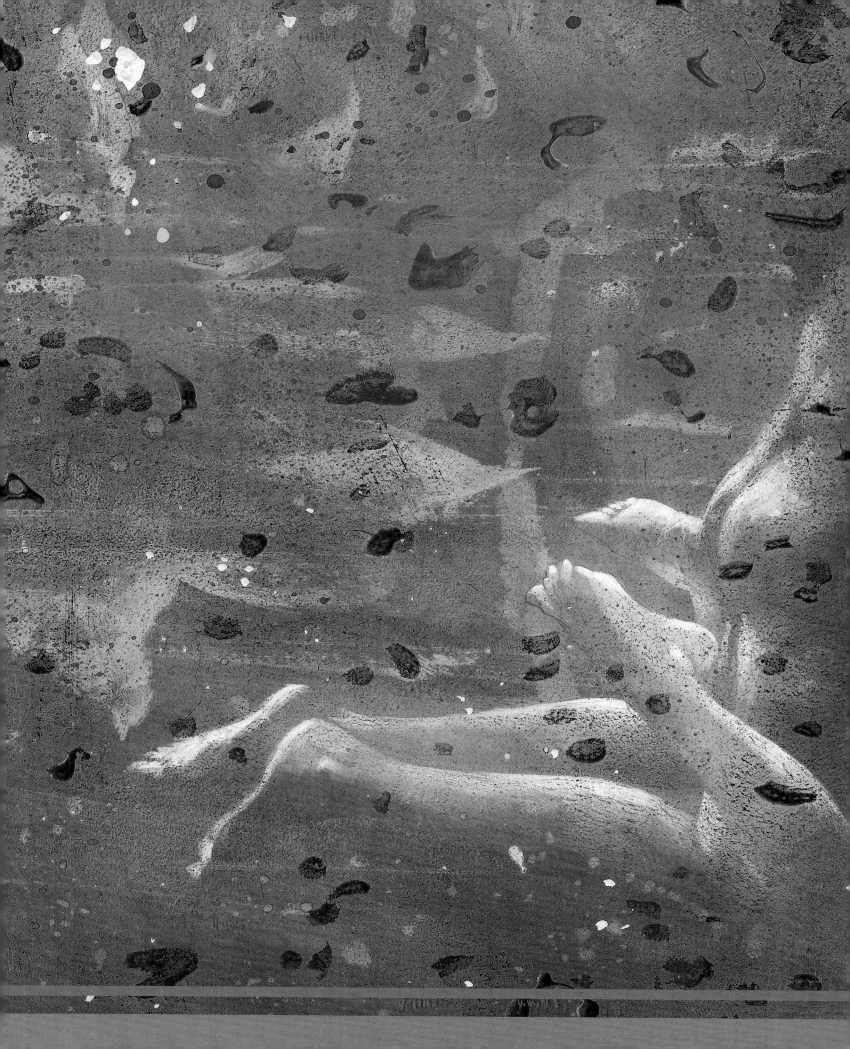

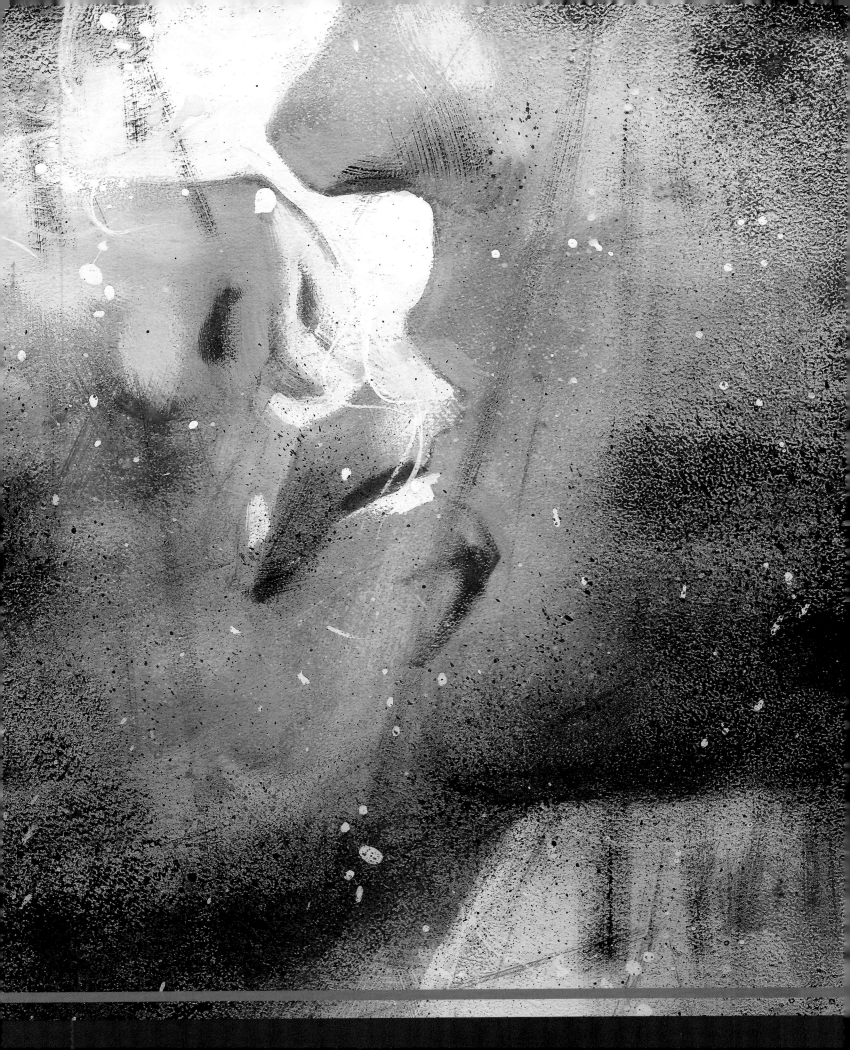

How to Kiss

Some say that you cannot set down a prescribed order for when to touch, kiss, scratch with the nails, or squeeze with the fingers during the act of love, because all these things should be done however they arise before sexual union. Once intercourse begins, striking the body and making noises find their proper place. However, Vatsyayana disagrees: anything can take place at any time. Love doesn't care about time and order.

When two lovers first have sex, kissing and these other things should be done moderately, not taking too long, alternating one with the other. After the first time, this is reversed. Lovers can take all the time they want to kindle their desire, and to that end they can mix up any kind of foreplay they want.

Kissing applies to the following parts of the body: forehead, eyes, cheeks, throat, breasts, lips, and inside the mouth. People of the Lat country kiss on more places: to the hip joint and knees, the arms and navel. Vatsyayana thinks that this may be their custom, justified by the intensity of their passion during lovemaking, but that kissing these parts of the body shouldn't become a general practice here.

For young girls there are three kinds of kisses: a light peck or nominal kiss, a throbbing kiss, and a touching kiss. When the girl only brushes her lips against her lover's, without actively kissing him, that is the nominal kiss. If she sets aside her bashfulness enough to respond to her lover's kiss by moving her lower lip but not her upper, that's a throbbing kiss. If she comes to the point that she takes her lover's hands and sticks out her tongue a little over her lower lip, that is a touching kiss.

Writers describe four other kinds of kissing: the straight kiss, the bent kiss, the turned kiss, and the pressed kiss.

Bringing your lips into direct contact with your lover's is the straight kiss. If your faces are at an angle to each other, that is the bent kiss. If you hold your lover's face tilted up with your hands while running your lips up and down hers, that is the turned kiss. Finally, if you forcefully push your lips onto hers, that is the pressed kiss. (One could add an even more forceful version, the hard-pressed kiss, which works this way: parting her lips with your fingers, you press your tongue hard against the lower lip, along with strong pressure from your own lips.)

A LOVER'S BET

You can place a coy wager on which of you will seize the other's lips first. If the man wins, the woman can pretend to cry, beating him off with fluttering hands and begging for another chance. If she should lose a second time, she can pull away, acting even more upset. Then, when her lover is off guard or asleep, she sneaks up and bites his lower lip with her teeth, holding on tight enough that he can't slip away. Then she can mock him, crowing and dancing around, pretending to have won a victory. This is a kissing wager, but the same game can be played with biting, scratching, or striking each other — these versions, however, are reserved for lovers who are full of great passion.

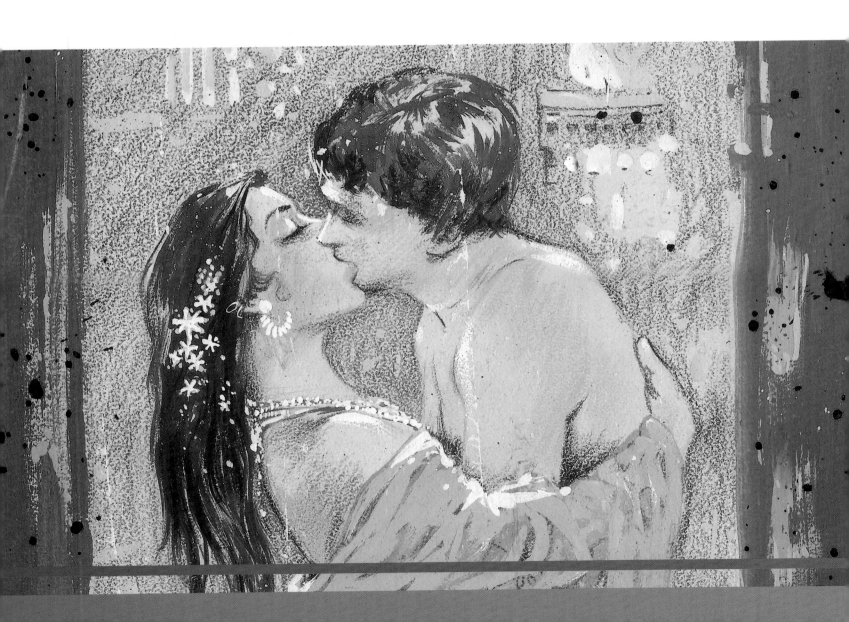

When a man and woman exchange a kiss where he takes her upper lip and she takes his lower lip, this is an upper-lip kiss. When one of you encloses both of your lover's lips between your own, that is termed 'the clasping kiss'. (A woman only gives such a kiss from a man without a moustache, however.) In the middle of this kiss, if one of you inserts a tongue to touch the other's teeth, tongue, or palate, that is called 'tongue fighting'. During this practice the bared teeth can be passed over your lover's lips, also.

Different kinds of kisses are appropriate for different parts of the body, varying from soft and moderate to pressing and contracted.

When a woman gazes at the face of her lover and wakes him with a light kiss to show her desire for sex, that is called a 'kiss that kindles love'. If she comes up on him with a kiss while he is doing business, or in the middle of a quarrel, or while he is paying attention to something else altogether, so that she can get his attention, it is known as a 'kiss that turns away'.

When a man coming home late at night kisses his beloved, who is asleep in bed, to show her his desire for lovemaking, it is called a 'kiss that awakens'. When this happens she may pretend to be asleep when he comes home, so that she may discover his intention and obtain respect from him.

When anyone kisses the reflection of the person he or she loves in a mirror, in water, or on a wall, it is called a 'kiss showing intention'. If this kiss happens with the beloved in the room — it may be a kiss given to a child sitting in one's lap or to a painting or statue — it is called a 'transferred kiss'. A man might kiss a woman's hand at the theater, or her foot if she is sitting down. A woman in turn may place her head on a man's thigh while bathing him, as if she feels sleepy, and then give a little kiss to the thigh to inflame him. These are called 'demonstrative kisses'.

There is also a verse that applies: 'Whatever may be done by one lover to the other, the same should be returned — if the woman kisses him he should kiss her back, if she bites, scratches, or strikes him he should do these back in kind.'

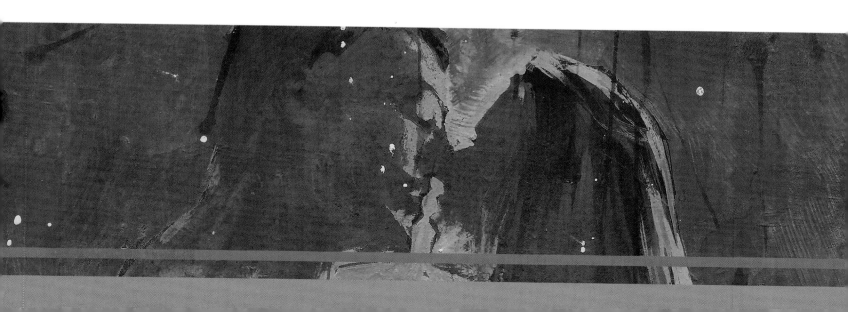

LEAVING YOUR MARK

During intense lovemaking there is scratching with the nails, which is done on the following occasions: the first union, before leaving home on a long journey, returning from the journey, at the time when two angry lovers are reconciled, and when the woman is drunk.

If a person is about to set off on a journey and leaves three or four marks on the lover's body, usually on the breast or thigh, this is called a 'token of remembrance'. It takes the form of long, straight scratches rather close together. But digging in one's nails is not a regular practice except among the most intense and passionate couples, who often accompany it with biting.

Using the nails falls into eight categories:

Sounding: This is pressing your nails into the chin, breasts, lower lip, the lower half of the body below the navel, or the thighs. Pressure is soft, so that no scratch or other mark is left, but the nails make a sound — thus the name of 'sounding' or pressing with the nails. This practice is used on young girls when they are being shampooed by their lovers — or when the man wants to scare them a little.

Half moon and circle: A curved mark left on the skin is called a half moon. It becomes a circle if there are two curves facing each other. The half moon is usually made on the neck or breasts. The circle is usually made around the navel, on the indentation of the buttocks, or at the hip joint.

Line: A straight mark left by the nails is called a line and can be done anywhere on the body.

Tiger claw: If the line curves over the surface of the breast it becomes a tiger claw.

Peacock's foot: It takes great skill to draw a curved line on the breast using all five fingers. When accomplished correctly, this is known as a peacock's foot, and the reason for making it is to win praise.

Rabbit jump: When five marks are left close together on the breast, usually bunched up around the nipple, this is known as a rabbit jump.

Blue lotus: A mark can also be left on the breast or hip that looks like the outline of a blue lotus leaf and is given that name.

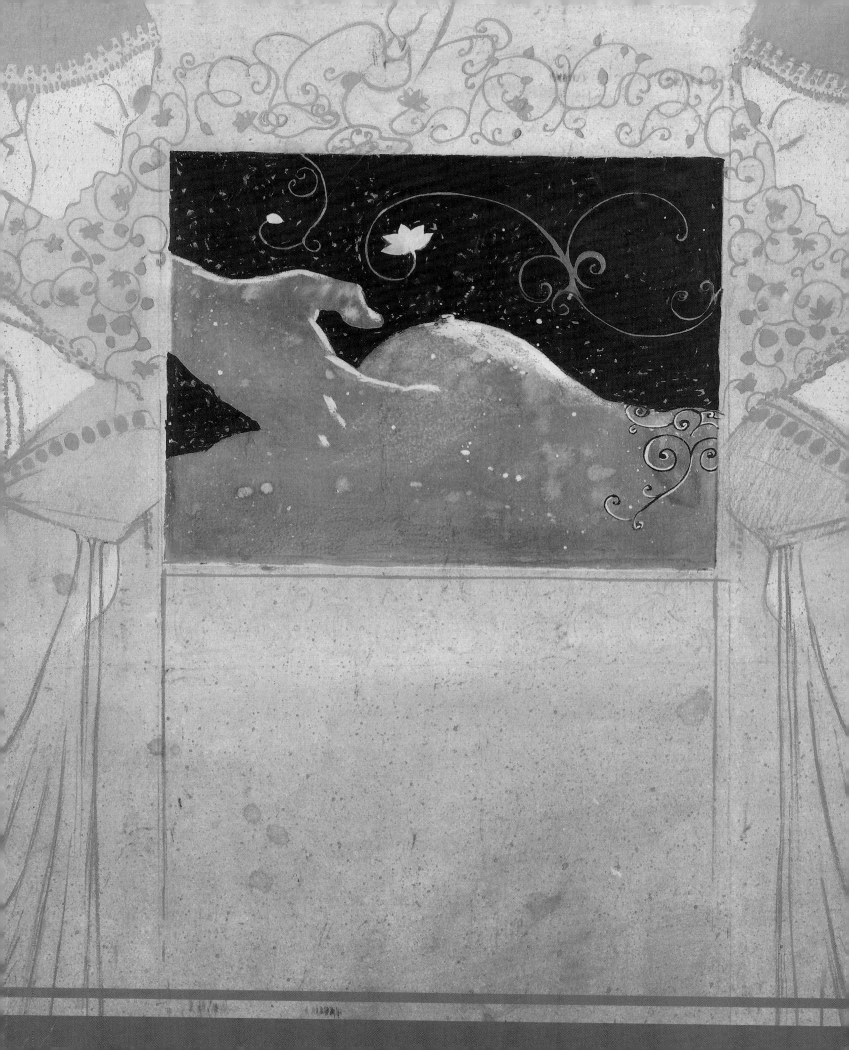

BATTLE OF THE SEXES

Because love is so contrary and so often leads to arguments, sexual intercourse takes on the appearance of a fight. When two lovers hit each other, there are some special places prescribed: head, shoulders, between the breasts, the back, mid-section and sides of the body. Striking is of four kinds: using the back of the hand, the fingers a little contracted together, the fist, and the open palm.

Since being hit causes pain, various sounds accompany the sexual fight, such as hissing, cooing, and crying. Besides these, there are also words having a meaning, such as 'mother', and those that are expressive of wanting the blows to stop, asking for less or more, wanting to break free, or expressing pain or praise. One might also make sounds like a dove, cuckoo, pigeon, parrot, bee, sparrow, flamingo, duck or quail — each is found in use occasionally.

In such a fight, blows with the fist should be given on the woman's back while she is sitting on the man's lap, and she should give the same in return, abusing the man as if she were angry, also making cooing and weeping sounds. During intercourse the space between the breasts should be struck with the back of the hand, slowly at first, and then becoming more intense with mounting excitement, until the end.

Some verses apply here:

'The two male characteristics are said to be roughness and impetuosity, while the female characteristics are frailty, tenderness, sensitivity, and an inclination to turn away from unpleasant things. During the excitement of passion, the opposite characteristics may appear, but they do not last long and soon after a person regains his or her natural state.'

'Such practices (of fighting and inflicting pain) cannot be fully numbered or set down with rules. Once passion begins, these acts arise spontaneously from the excitement of the parties involved.'

'Such acts are as hard to define as dreams. A horse going full tilt will drive blindly on, regardless of holes, ditches, or posts in his way. Likewise, a loving couple can become blind in the act of intercourse and impetuously proceed without the least regard for excess. Not all practices are suitable all the time — they have their own time and place. A man, knowing his own strength and the tenderness or strength of the woman, should proceed accordingly when it is appropriate.'

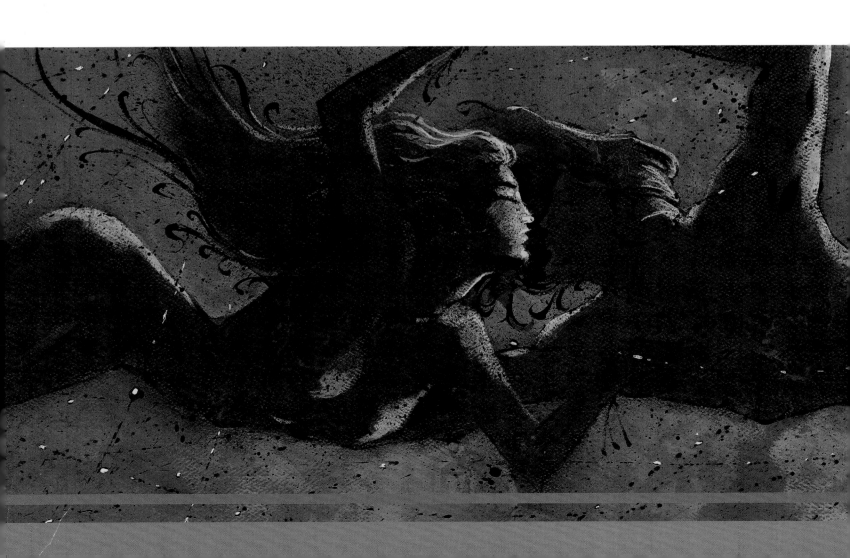

THE WOMAN PLAYING THE MAN'S PART

If a woman notices that a man is getting tired out during sex and isn't coming to orgasm, she can assist him, after asking permission, by turning him onto his back and taking over his role. She can also do this out of curiosity, either her own or the man's, or for the sake of novelty.

There are two basic approaches to this reversal. She can slide into the man's role during intercourse without interrupting the pleasure they are both receiving, or she can adopt the man's role from the outset. Chaffing him, she should say, 'You laid me down and wore me out with your thrusts, now I am turning the tables and doing the same to you.' Poised over him with flowers hanging loose from her hair, panting and smiling by turns, she begins to do the man's work.

What is meant by the man's work is as follows: As the woman is lying in his bed, he distracts her with conversation while quietly undoing her undergarments. When she protests, he overcomes her with kisses. Once he is erect, he touches and manipulates her in various places. If the woman is shy and it's the first time they have come together, the man puts his hands between her thighs, which she will probably keep closed, and if she is a young girl, he would first get his hands on her breasts, which she would probably cover with her own hands; he would likewise touch her under the armpits and on her neck. If she is an experienced woman, however, he can do whatever is agreeable either to him or to her, and whatever is fitting for the occasion. After this he takes hold of her hair and chin for the purpose of kissing her. At this point, if she is a young girl, she will become bashful and close her eyes. Anyhow he should gather from the action of the woman what things would be pleasing to her during intercourse.

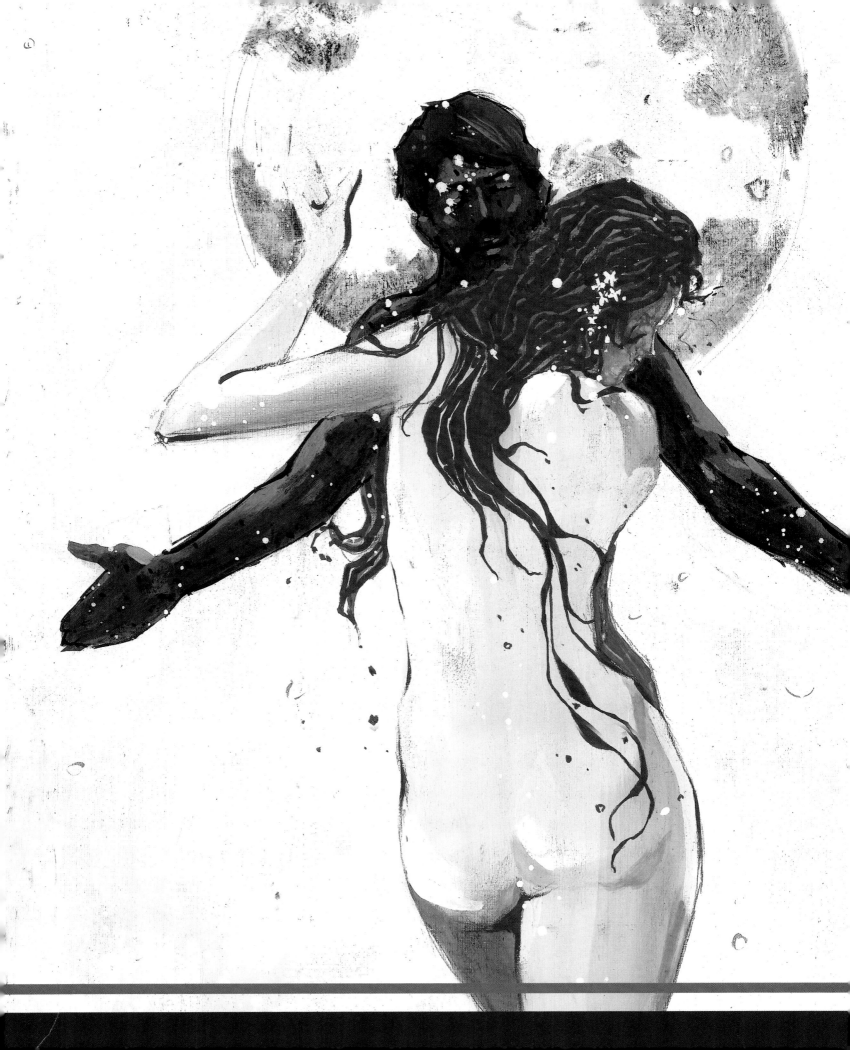

Here Suvarnanabha says that while a man is doing to the woman what he likes best during congress, he should always make a point of pressing those parts of her body on which she turns her eyes. The signs of enjoyment and satisfaction in a woman are as follows: her body relaxes, she closes her eyes, she puts aside all bashfulness and shows increased willingness to unite their two organs as closely together as possible. On the other hand, the signs of her lack of enjoyment and of failing to be satisfied are as follows: she shakes her hands, she does not let the man get up, feels dejected, bites the man, kicks him, and continues to go on moving after the man has finished. To avoid this the man should rub the organ of the woman with his hand and fingers (as the elephant rubs anything with his trunk) before engaging in sex until it is softened, and after that is done he should proceed to put his penis into her.

When the woman is tired, she should place her forehead on that of her lover, and should thus take rest without disturbing the union of the organs, and when the woman has rested herself the man should turn round and begin the sex again.

A verse on the subject is as follows: 'Though a woman is reserved and keeps her feelings concealed; yet when she gets on the top of a man she shows all her love and desire. A man should gather from the actions of a woman what kind of disposition she has and in what way she likes to be enjoyed.'

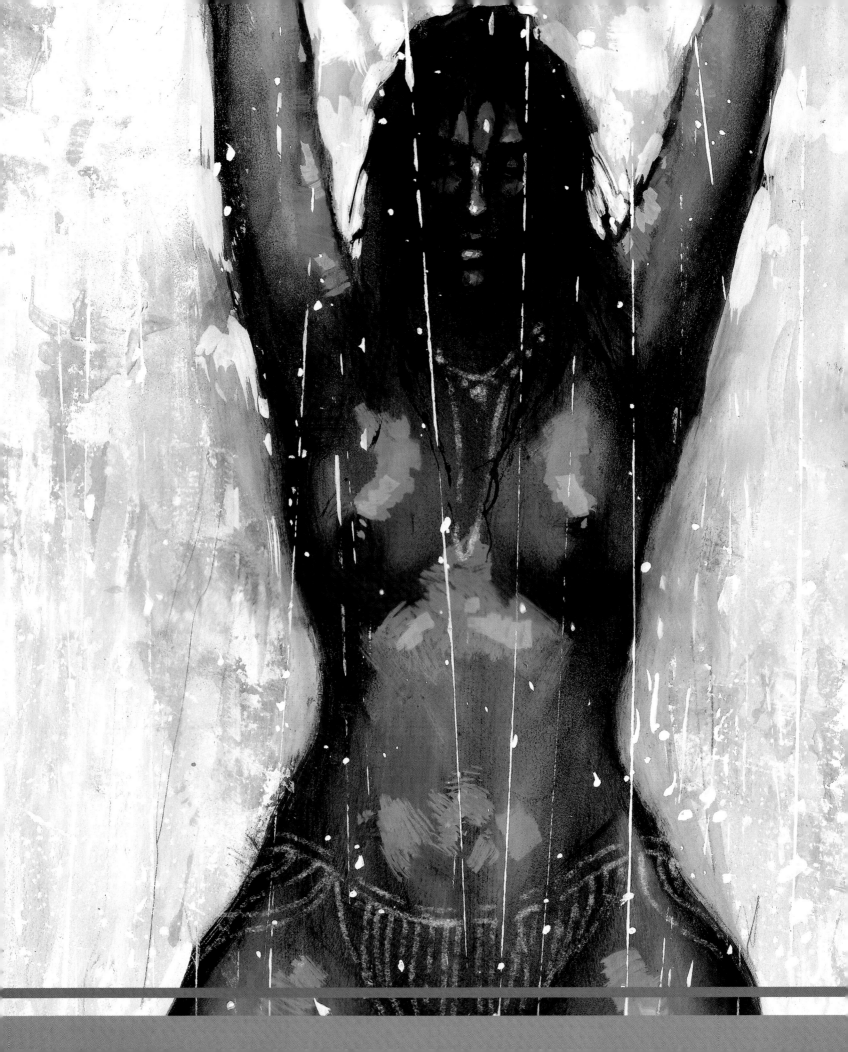

FOREPLAY

You ardent young men, don't forget foreplay! You are here to satisfy your woman. Listen to what she wants, to the way of her desire.

Some young men, overwhelmed by their own desire, forget the prelude and are surprised when the woman pushes them away later. But it's so delightful to kiss and caress and nibble at one another, exploring with your hand or mouth all the places of her body — her neck, breasts, stomach, down to the innermost curves. Being fulfilled, the woman can return your kisses and caresses wholeheartedly. Neglect no smallest part of her body. The man should make it his duty to discover them, and once found to show his lover the refined pleasures to be had there.

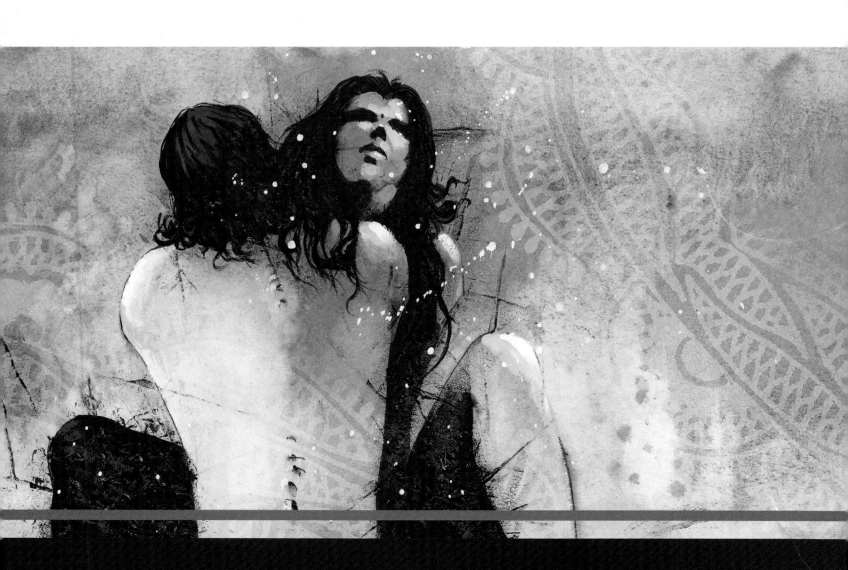

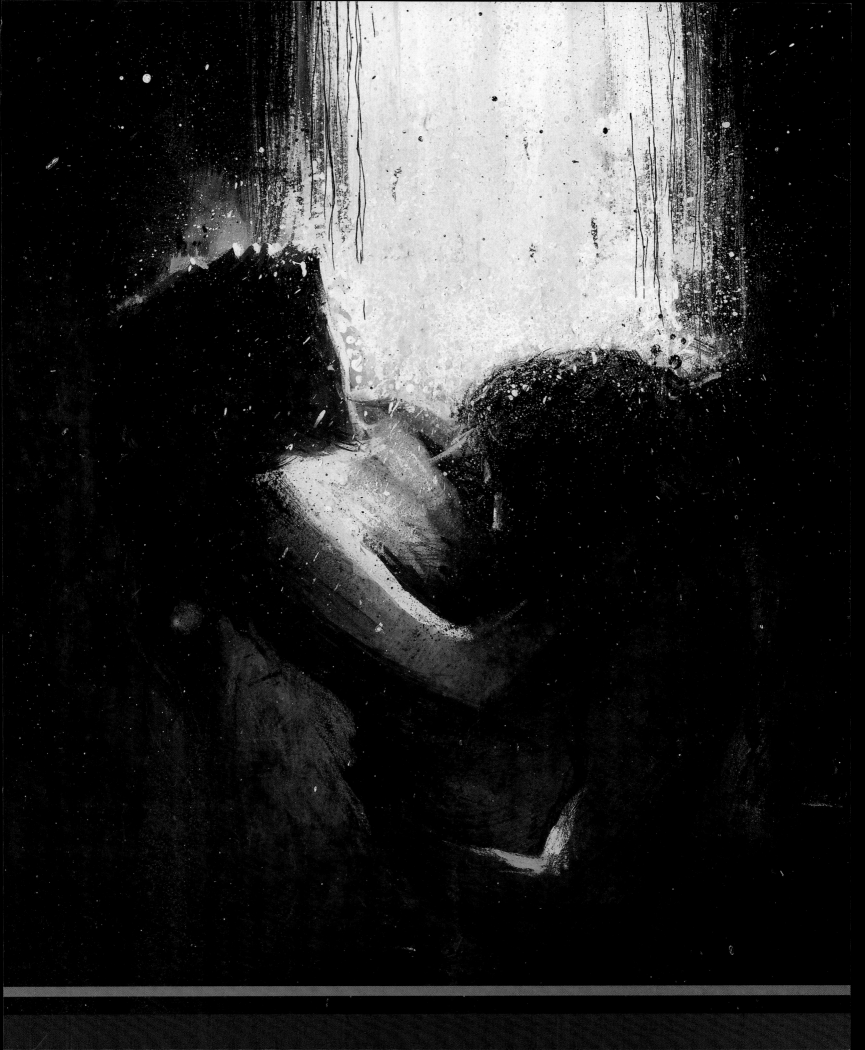

DIVINE LOVEMAKING

In primordial times the cosmos was ruled by darkness. The gods felt powerless to defeat the darkness until Indra was created, Indra the perfect male. He killed the arch-demon Vritra, and thus an orderly world was allowed to grow in place of chaos. Indra is beautiful like the sun, and like the sun he burns ardently. Only a perfect woman, called Padmini, can satisfy him. A Padmini, with her thousand virtues, is one in ten million. Still, you other women, don't despair! With patience and care any woman can perfect the position in which Indra's wife makes love, resting on her back with her knees drawn to her chest and her feet resting on her thighs. Then the man and woman can share an encounter with the divine essence which promises fertility and love.

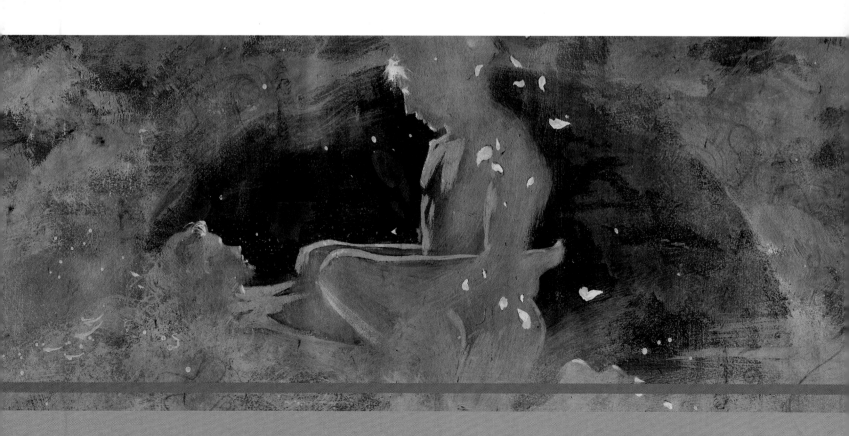

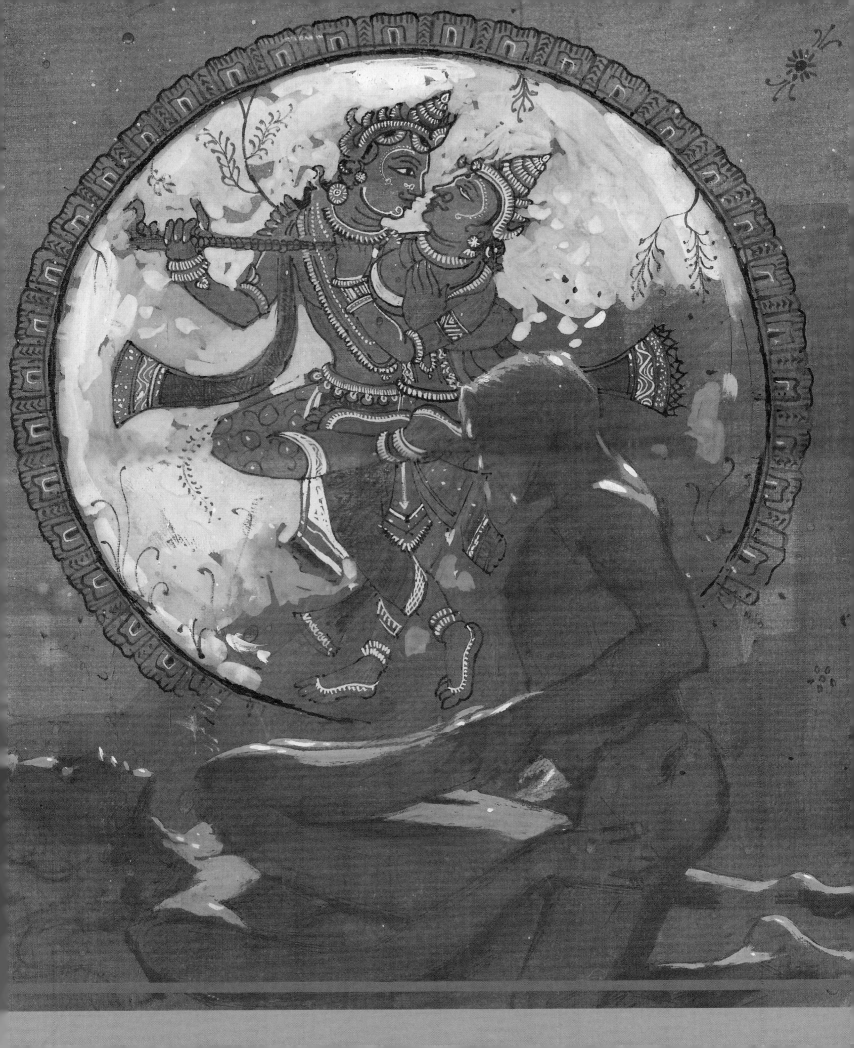

THE STROKES OF LOVE

A man can make love with his penis using ten different strokes:

- Grasping his penis in his hand he can move it in circles inside the vagina. This is called 'churning' (Mantha).

- He can strike sharply downward into the vagina. This is called 'the double-edged sword' (Hula).

- With the woman's hips raised up on a pillow, he can push in a rising motion. This is called 'rubbing' (Avamardana).

- He can press his penis excitedly into her womb and hold it there. This is called 'pressing' (Piditaka).

- He can pull out completely and then re-enter with a hard stroke. This is called 'buffeting' (Nirghata).

- He can put continuous pressure to one side of the vagina. This is called 'the boar's blow' (Varahaghata).

- He can thrust wildly in all directions like a bull tossing his horns. This is called 'the bull's blow' (Vrishaghata).

- He can quiver inside her vagina, as usually happens just before orgasm. This is called 'sparrow's play' (Chatakavilasa).

- He can give an involuntary shudder inside her, such as a man makes at orgasm. This is called 'the jewel case' (Samputa).

- He can give a gentle stroke forward, which may be varied in depth and speed. This is the only position known as 'natural' (Upasnipta). It comes without instruction even to a cowherd in the fields and allows for full pleasure to the woman's clitoris. It also gives lovemaking a subtlety, rhythm, and spontaneity that the other positions lack in one way or another.

But no two women are alike, and you are always advised to adapt your stroke and rhythm to the emotions your partner is feeling at the time.

THE ABANDONED WOMAN

A deserted wife mourns the happy times when her husband showered her with caresses. To get him to return to her, she prays to the sacred cow Kamadhenu. Suddenly the man returns with a tale. He had a dream of Kamadhenu; the cow had his wife's face, and in it he once again saw her beauty, except that her lips trembled and her eyes were glistening with tears. Repentant, the husband throws himself at his wife's feet. When she forgives him, he embraces her so ardently that she almost suffocates. He hugs and kisses her breasts, her thighs. Thanking the divine Kamadhenu for opening his eyes, the husband turns his penis around inside the woman's delicious vagina — a divine reunion which takes the name 'churning the milk'.

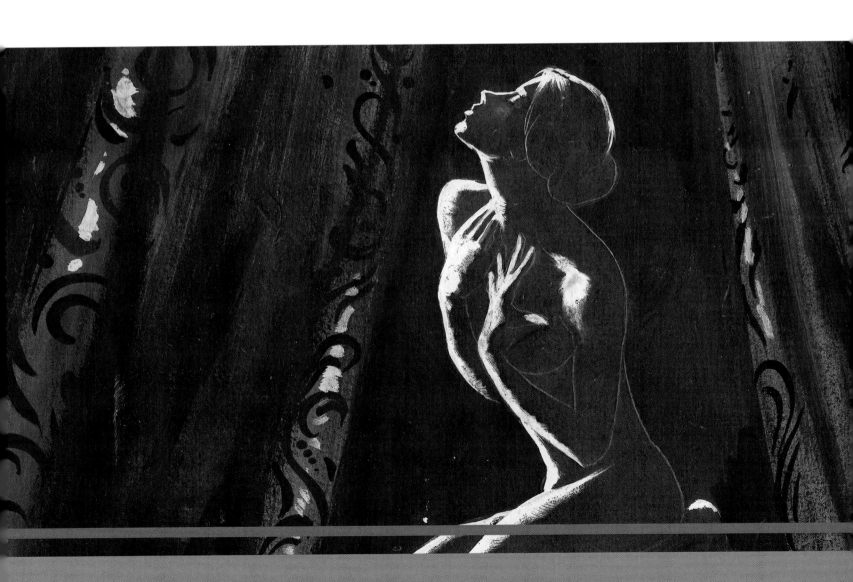

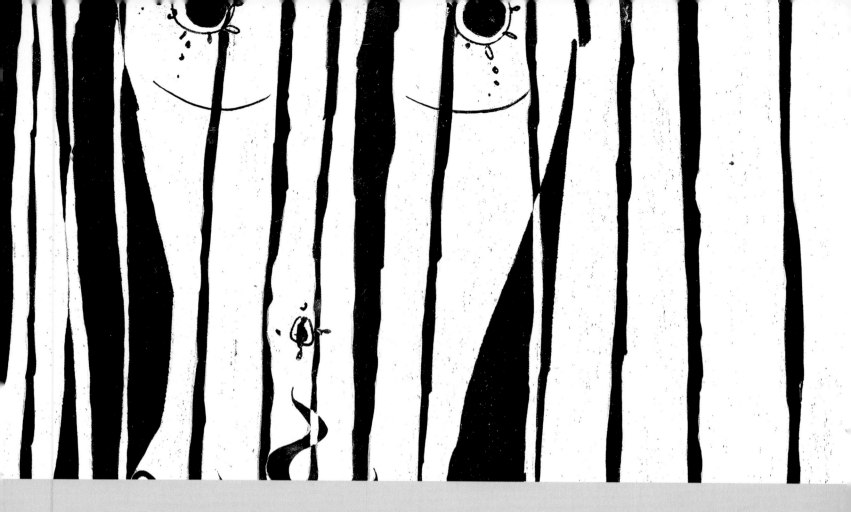

THE ROYAL HAREM

Nowhere is as poorly guarded as a harem, and no women are more accessible than the wives of the king. An enterprising young man can choose any number of ways to get inside. Hidden in a barrel or masquerading as a maid, he can easily get past the lazy sentries and overworked servants. Another possibility is to take a potion that will make him invisible — but the outcome of this is uncertain.

Runaway Passion

It's a lazy hot afternoon; even the flies are asleep. A young engaged couple manage to sneak away for a secret rendezvous. They are refined and charming, skilled in the art of love. They kiss in all the ways they've been taught: straight on, to the side, lips pressed hard together, tongues fighting . . . but wait! They get so carried away that they forget these refined ways. All at once they are ripping off each other's sweat-soaked silk clothes. They roll naked on the cold tile floor like dogs! Mouth to mouth, eyes gazing at each other, limbs intertwined — you can hardly tell one from the other. Like mixing sesame seeds and rice, their genitals mingle and meet. It seems the charming engaged couple have celebrated their wedding night in advance!

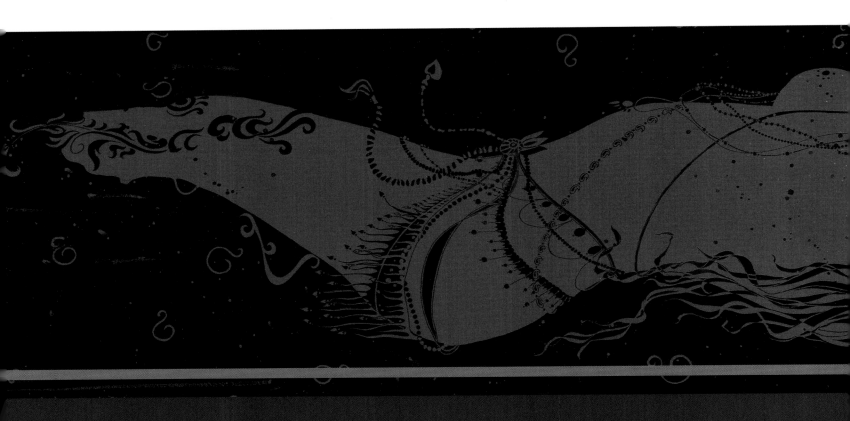

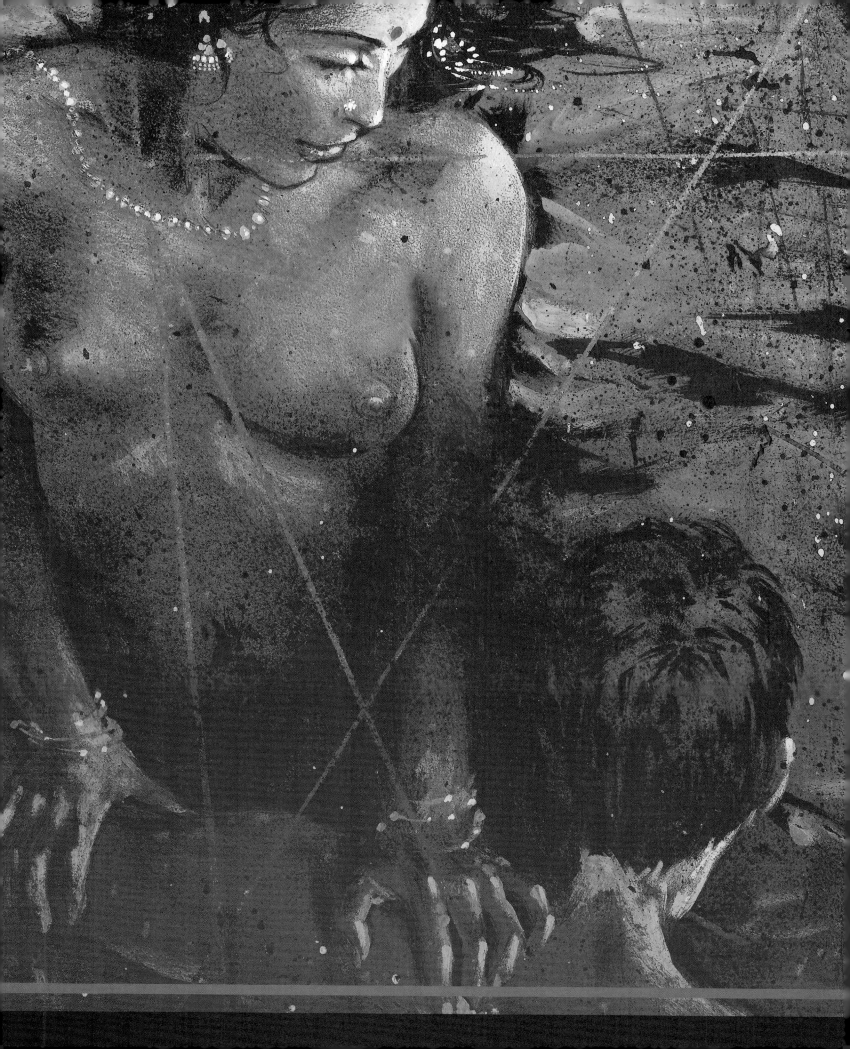

MIDNIGHT YEARNING

The lover kneels beside the bed of a girl sleeping in modest beauty under the moonlight. He wakes her gently with a kiss to the forehead. She smiles, keeping her eyelids closed. The lover grabs her around the hips and slides her onto his lap. The beauty provocatively spreads her legs; this inflames him to enter her. Her ankle bracelets tinkle seductively. The lover wants to possess what she has revealed, then and there. But she wants to tease him a bit more, and when he protests, she silences him by putting one of her delicate feet over his mouth. He nibbles at her toes one at a time, making her coo like a dove. She coos so loud that she wakes up the morning dove, who begins to answer her — this makes her laugh. Just enough diversion for the eager lover to get his way; with a single swift stroke, he enters her.

Thus those who know love say sweet words while approaching a woman with a penis erect as a pole. With one fast motion they plunge into her, piercing her vagina and uniting their bodies. This is called Madandhvaja — the flat of Eros.

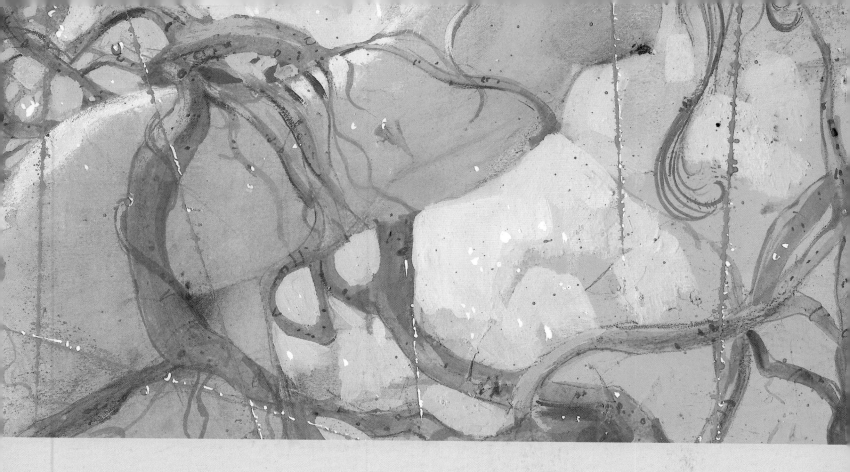

SEDUCED BY A COBRA

He's the ideal catch: rich, educated, and respectable. Only behind closed doors does his wife know this paragon's weakness. As brave and forceful as he can be playing games, he has no energy for the game of love. But she has a plan. She fixes all kinds of amorous potions, blending milk and sugar, medicinal roots and licorice for him to drink, and rice with sparrow's eggs to eat. Then before going to bed she perfumes her body with luscious oils. Her skillful caresses begin to interest his penis.

Suddenly, with a hiss she draws back. Coiling her body up like a snake, she slithers away and buries herself in the pillows, hiding her vagina from him. Her husband didn't expect this reversal. Aroused and ready, his penis has to have her! Blindly it reaches for her vagina. This is the coupling of the cobra.

LOTUS POSITION

The woman lies on her back with her legs raised. With her ankles crossed, she chains them behind her husband's neck and grasps her toes while he makes love to her. This is Padma, the lotus, a delightful position.

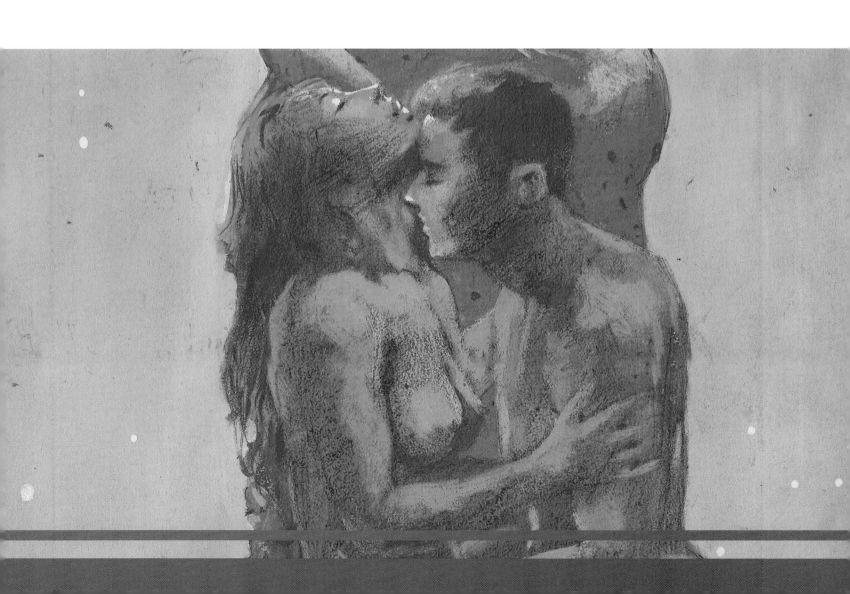

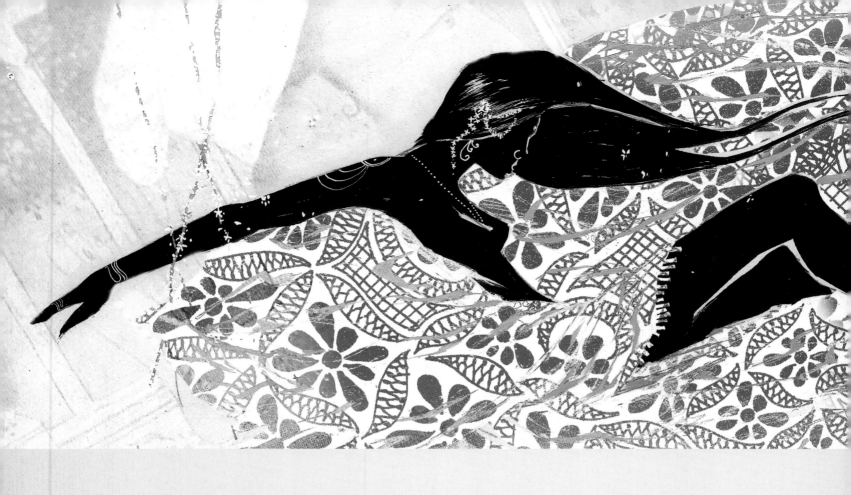

SIREN OF THE SEA

She makes love like a sea-woman, like the whole ocean. Her hair glistening with sweat, she curls up like seaweed in her lover's arms. Her teeth are as lustrous as the pearls she's wearing. The fisherman tries to nibble at the little pink fish of her tongue, but it quickly darts away. He takes a deep breath and dives toward her vagina and its soft glisten. A cruel bite brings him up again with a cry. Her teeth hold his flesh like a moray eel! Imitating the octopus, she wraps him up in her tentacles and drags him down to the abyss. He is delighted to drown! The beautiful siren finally surrenders. He straddles her lifted thighs and enters, keeping her firmly positioned with his knees. In the ocean of pleasure they are like the two halves of that lovely shellfish, the conch.

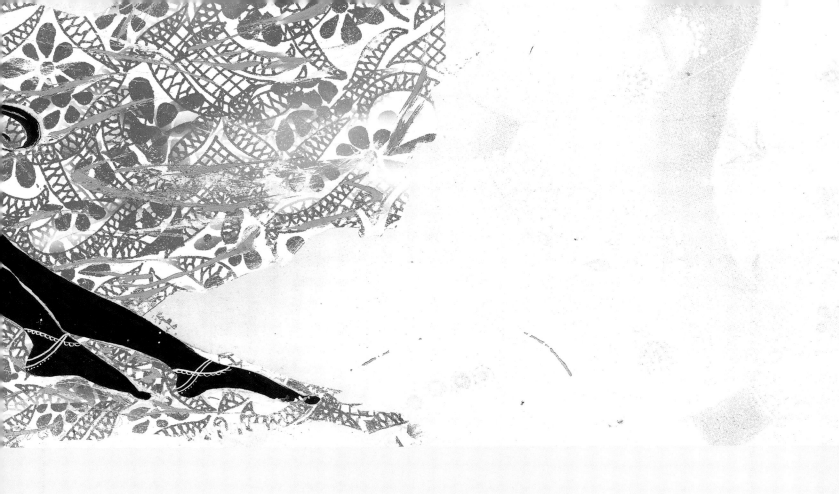

THE SWEETEST REVENGE

Everything seems set up for love: perfume in the air, flower petals strewn over the sheets. But these two are stand-offish and keep their distance. Oh, they aren't lovers at all — they're deceived spouses! Their unfaithful partners are attracted to each other. So these two are meeting to talk it out. The betrayed wife starts to cry. The deceived husband thinks it's only his duty to console her. Strangely, he had always thought she was a little too fat for him, but now he's aroused. He wipes her tears away with a gentle caress. She gives him a polite kiss in return, so as not to be in his debt. Such a nice man, too. Pretty soon it's a contest in courtesy: they cuddle, tickle, embrace each other. Suddenly he's as erect as a mast; he seizes her and enters. He pounds and polishes her like a pestle. What sweet revenge!

AMAZON

Is it the full moon? You don't recognize her anymore, this sweet, devoted wife. Tonight she's like an Amazon, immense and fierce. She wants to be on top, a proud warrior ready to conquer! Offering her belly like a wolf, she gives you no choice but to surrender; she's going to tame you. There's no use resisting her arrogant breasts, her flat belly, her muscled thighs, and greedy mouth. They are so many weapons tonight. Your weapon is more modest, but it's ready for the fight. She grasps it and sits over you, legs tucked up. She sucks you into her until you cry out. Then a surprise talent — she begins to swivel on your penis like a top, with you as her pivot.

On top: There are three famous lovemaking styles for the woman when she takes the man's position:

68

- She can steal a trick from the mare and hold your penis inside her like a vise, gripping, squeezing, and stroking it. If she keeps it inside for a hundred heartbeats, this is known as Sarndamsha, the Tongs.
- She can crouch in a sitting position over you, revolving her vagina around your penis while you help her by arching your back. This is called Bhrarnara, the Bee.
- She can sway in wide circles over you with her body, making a figure eight. This is known as Prenkholita, the Swing.

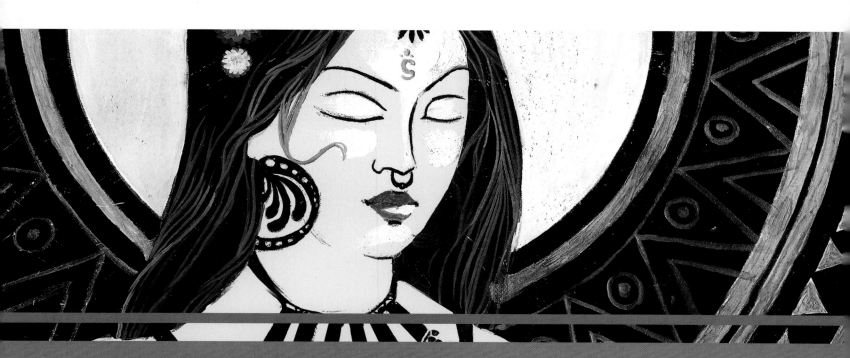

THE PROFESSIONAL

The fame of a certain courtesan from the land of Andra has spread far and wide. This is because she makes love with consummate artistry. It's rumored that she always climbs on top of the man, unlike the mare. When he's relaxed and tamed, smothered in caresses, she abruptly seizes him inside her. His penis is squeezed deep in her vagina, all but strangling it — thus the perfection of the Mare's Stroke. Men want to buy the secret from her; so do women, many of them respectable wives. But the courtesan of Andra doesn't need your money; she's already rich. The only affection she has to give is for Babu, her baby elephant.

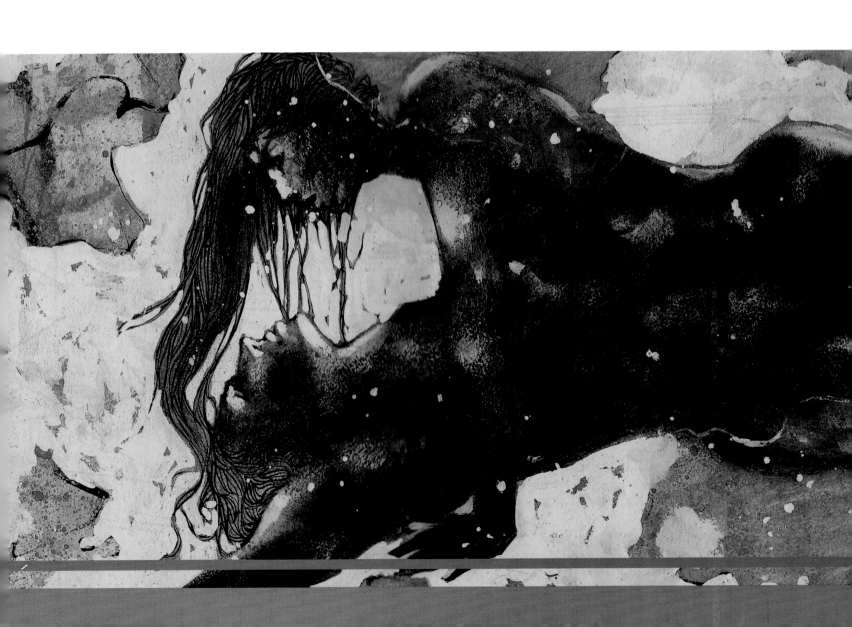

THE GENTLEMAN AND THE SWING

There's a refined gentleman of the town, a man of taste. He has two swings in his garden. One goes back and forth, the other whirls in a circle. He whiles away the hours talking to his friends of an evening, but after they're gone, he sometimes gets in the swings. He goes from one to the other, and sometimes the whole thing makes his head swim.

But his favorite swing doesn't have rope or plank or pillow. No, it's his skillful courtesan, who is passionate in her lovemaking. She greets him decorated with pearls and gold, a sheer veil the only thing that hides her modesty. Stretching her arms out for him, they know the night ahead will be a long one. They reopen all 64 chapters of the book of love, ending with the swing. She sits on his lap with her legs raised. With one hand he steadies her, with the other he caresses her breasts while she swings back and forth, faster and faster, until he is in ecstasy.

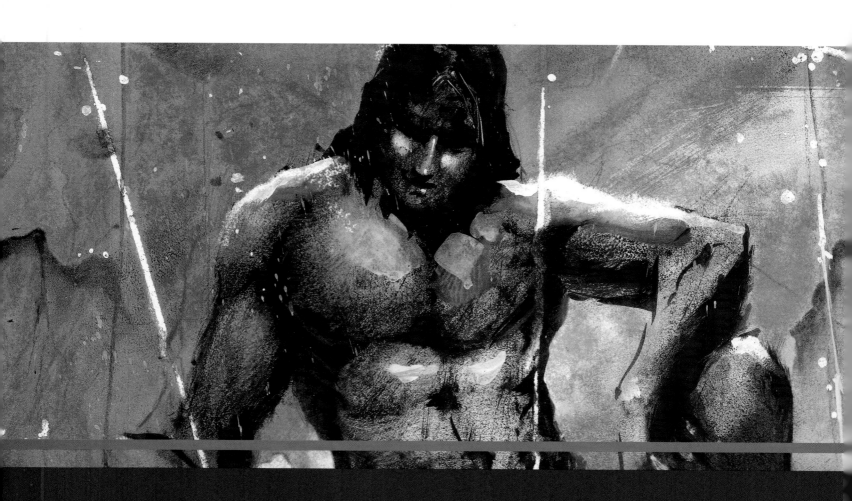

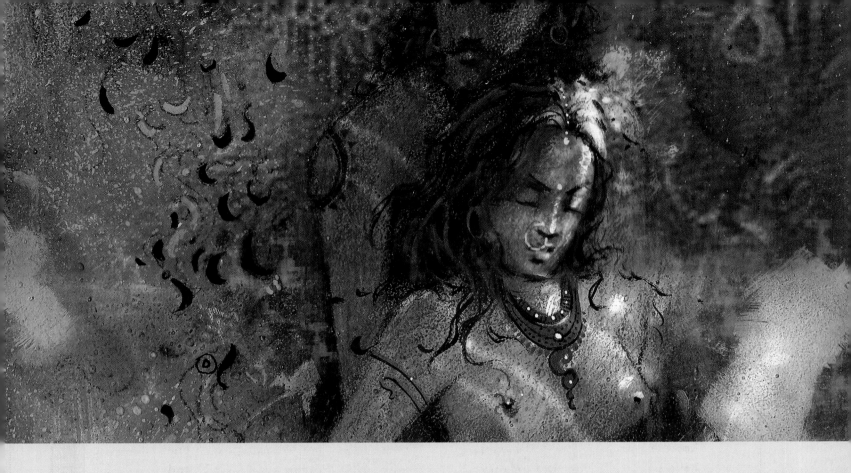

In the Den of the Tigress

The lover has been away for a few weeks, but now at last he's back. The marks his lovemaking has left on his mistress's body have long faded away. For some reason this intimidates him. What if she's no longer his? She looks more radiant than he can remember, and suddenly he wonders if another man has been there. A cloud darkens his mind. Could she really have deceived him? As if reading his mind, she begins to make love like a tigress, digging her nails into his shoulders. He feels it like animal claws, like a peacock's talons, a swollen insect bite, a stabbing cloud of blows. She uses her teeth and nails like a wildcat! But then the lover, being cunning too, slides his hand between her thighs. He caresses her delicately until the tigress turns into a purring, contented kitty cat.

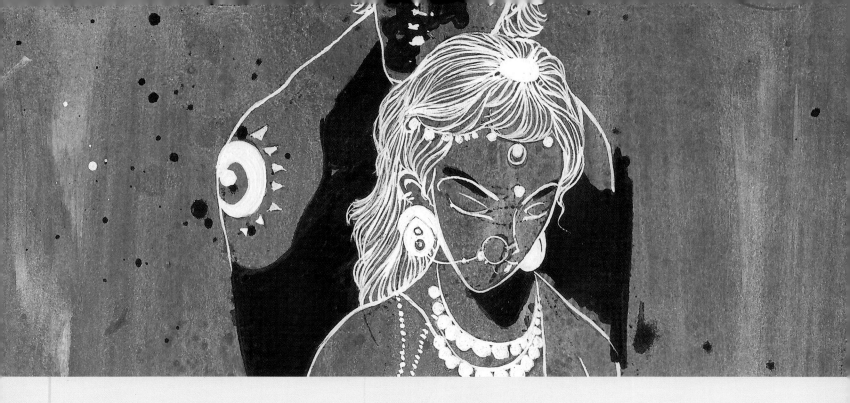

THE ELEPHANT

Have you ever marveled at the elephant? He combines such strength and delicacy. Consider his trunk, so powerful that it can uproot a tree, yet so delicate that it can curl around an object gently or barely skim over it with a touch. Keep this in mind when you meet those women who are intimidated or surprised by the size of a man's penis. Some men approach this problem as if the elephant is some kind of mythical rival. The knowing lover doesn't care a fig about rivals, whether men, women, or animals. He can't touch her with his trunk, after all! But it doesn't matter. Instead, he lifts his lover up and turns her around. Inhaling her intoxicating scent, he uses his penis to stroke the inside of her thighs, gently brushing her vagina. She appreciates how vigorous he becomes. Tonight, just for her, he is Hastica, the elephant.

Position: While your mistress lies face down with her forehead and breasts to the bed, raising up her buttocks you slide your penis into her vagina. This is called Aibha, the Elephant.

TYPES OF INTERCOURSE

When a man and woman who have been in love with each other for some time come together overcoming great difficulty, or when one of them returns from a journey or is reconciled after a quarrelsome separation, then their sex is called 'loving intercourse'. It is carried on according to the liking of the lovers and for as long as they choose.

When two people come together while their love is still in its infancy, their intercourse is called the 'intercourse of love to come'.

When a man has intercourse because he is excited through various ways such as kissing and fondling, etc., or when a man and woman come together though in reality they are both attached to different people, their sex is then called 'intercourse of artificial love'. At this time all the ways and means mentioned in the art of love should be used.

When a man, from the beginning to the end of the intercourse, though having connection with the woman, thinks all the time that he is enjoying another one whom he loves, it is called the 'intercourse of transferred love'.

Intercourse between a man and a female servant, or with a woman of a caste lower than his own, lasting only until the desire is satisfied, is called 'intercourse like that of eunuchs'. Here external touches, kisses, and manipulation are not to be employed.

The intercourse between a courtesan and a rustic, or between respectable citizens and the women of outlying villages and bordering countries, is called 'deceitful intercourse'.

The sex that takes place between two persons who are attached to one another, and which is done according to their own liking, is called 'spontaneous intercourse'.

LOVERS' SPATS

A woman who is very much in love with a man cannot bear to hear the name of her rival mentioned, or to have any conversation regarding her, or to be addressed by her name accidentally. If anything like this takes place, a great quarrel arises, and the woman cries, becomes angry, tosses her hair, strikes her lover, falls from her bed and, casting aside her garlands and ornaments, throws herself down on the ground.

At this time the man should attempt to reconcile her with conciliatory words; he should take her up carefully and place her back in bed. But she, not replying to his questions and with increased anger, should bend his head down by pulling his hair, and having kicked him once, twice, or thrice on his arms, head, bosom or back, she should then head for the door.

One authority, Dattaka, says that she should then sit angrily near the door and shed tears, but should not leave, because she would be found fault with for running out. After a time, when she thinks that the conciliatory words and actions of her lover have reached their utmost, she should then embrace him, talking to him with harsh and reproachful words, but at the same time showing a loving desire for sex.

If the woman is in her own house and begins quarreling with her lover, she should show how angry she is and walk out. Afterwards, the man having sent her pacifying gifts and tokens of remorse, she can return home and spend the night with him.

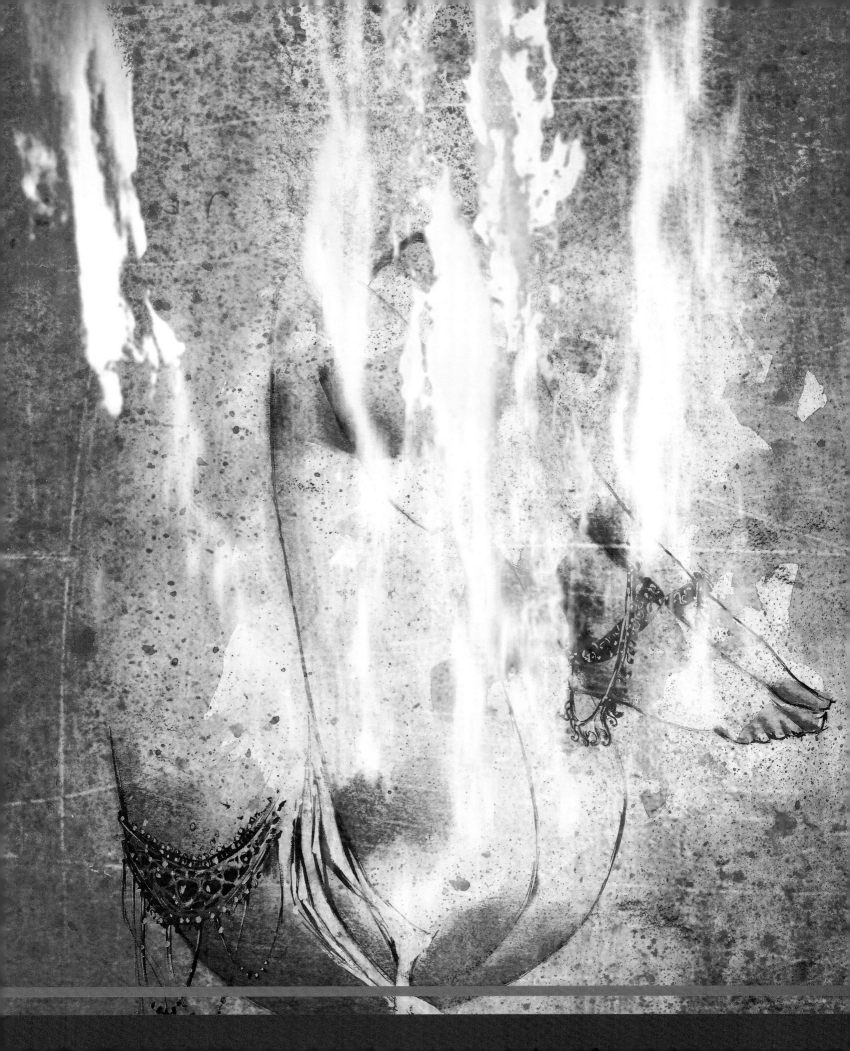

A Shy Bride

A man should win his new bride over by nurturing her confidence. Women, being of a tender nature, want tender beginnings. When they are forcefully approached by a man, who perhaps they have known only superficially, they may sometimes become haters of the sexual connection — and sometimes even haters of the male sex. The man should therefore approach the girl according to her own liking, doing whatever it takes to gradually win himself into her confidence. He can do various things to accomplish this.

He should favor the sexual position she feels most comfortable with, especially at the beginning, when the sex act doesn't last long.

Wrapping her in his arms is comforting and personal. If he has known her for a long time, he may embrace her with the light on, but if she is young and shy and they do not know each other well yet, he should embrace her in the dark.

Once the woman accepts his embrace, the man should gently feed her sweetmeat (in the original text, a betel leaf). If she doesn't take it, he should entreat her, and if she continues to resist, fall on his knees. It is a universal rule that, however bashful or angry a woman may be, she never disregards a man who kneels at her feet. When giving her this sweetmeat, the man should kiss her gently without making a sound.

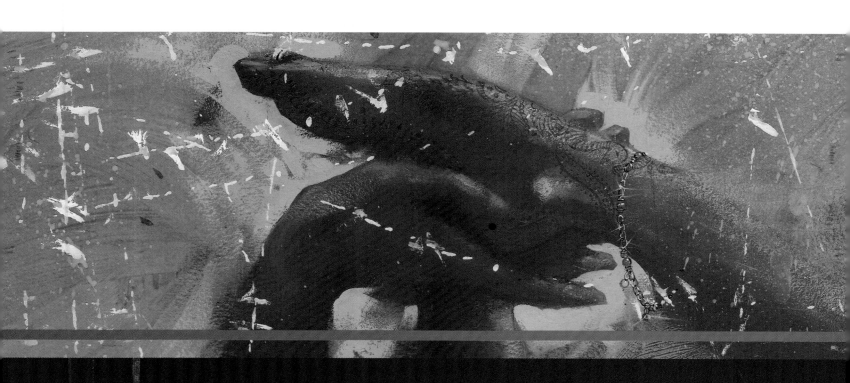

Next the man should get the woman to talk, which he does by asking her questions on topics that he knows nothing about — or pretends to know nothing — and which can be answered in a few words. If she won't speak, he shouldn't frighten her but instead keep repeating his questions over and over in a conciliatory manner.

If the man asks his bride if she desires him, she should modestly say nothing, but remain silent for a long time. If he keeps pressing the question, she should answer with a slight nod of the head. Once she gets to the point of returning his embrace, the man should lightly run his hands over her body. By and by he can place her in his lap and try more and more to gain her consent. If nothing works, he can try to frighten her by saying, 'If you don't give in I will scratch and bite you and then tell all my friends that you did them to yourself. Is that what you want?' This approach, among others, is how fear and confidence are instilled in children, and the man should try them to get the woman to give in to his desire.

At last, having won her over, he should enjoy her in such a way as not to frighten her, touching her entire body with his hands and kissing every part. He should also promise to be faithful forever and allay any fears she may have about other women.

A verse applies here: 'A man, acting on the inclinations of a girl, should try to gain her over so that she may love him and place her trust in him. A man doesn't succeed either by totally giving in to the woman or by opposing her. He should therefore adopt a middle course. A man who knows how to win a woman's love will be held in high honor and regard, but one who neglects a woman will be despised by her as a beast, ignorant of the ways of the female mind. Moreover, if a man forces himself on a shy girl, she becomes nervous, uneasy, and dejected. She will begin to hate the man who has taken advantage of her. If her love is never understood or returned, she will sink into despondency, becoming either a hater of men in general or a hater of her husband — then she will be driven into the arms of other men.'

DOES SHE LOVE HIM?

Now, a girl always shows her love by certain outward signs and actions, such as the following:

- She never looks the man in the face; she acts abashed when he looks at her.

- Under some pretext or other she lets him get a glimpse of her arms and legs.

- She secretly peeks at him though he has gone away from her side, hangs her head when she is asked some question by him, and answers with indistinct words and unfinished sentences.

- She spends long hours in his company.

- When he is at a distance, she talks to her friends in such a way as to attract his attention.

- If they are together, she makes excuses not to leave. She makes him look at various things or tell her long stories.

- She makes a show of kissing and embracing a small child sitting in her lap.

- She acts merry and sportive with her friends when the man is nearby.

- She confides in his friends, acting amiable and kind toward them, and listening closely when they talk about him.

- She avoids being seen by him when she isn't dressed with her make-up on.

- She wears anything he has given her all the time.

- Through her friends she gives him any small token, such as a ring or earring, that he has asked for.

- She becomes dejected when any other suitor is mentioned by her parents. She avoids the company of these prospective suitors and doesn't keep company with their friends.

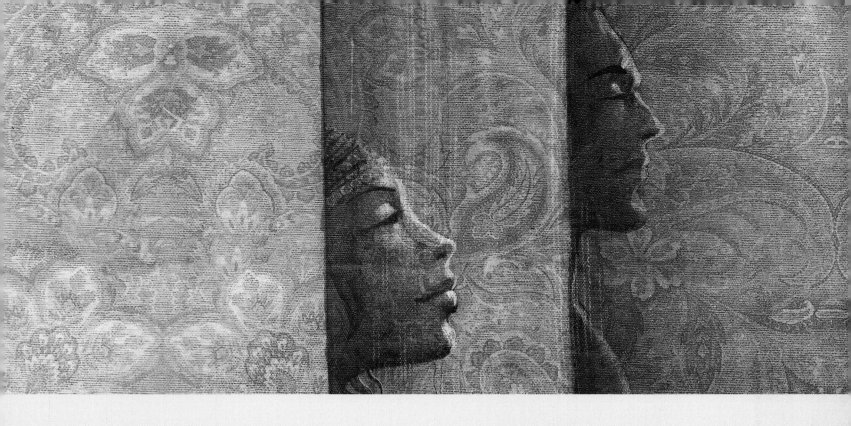

THE ART OF COYNESS

Old authors say that although the girl may love the man very much, she should not offer herself or make the first overtures, for a girl who does this loses her dignity and is liable to be scorned and rejected. But when the man shows his wish to be with her she should encourage him while showing no change in her demeanor, even when he embraces her. She should receive all the manifestations of his love as if she were ignorant of the state of his mind. When he tries to kiss her she should oppose him; when he begs to be allowed to have sex with her she should only let him touch her private parts — and this with considerable difficulty. Although importuned by him, she should not yield herself up to him as if of her own accord, but should resist his attempts to have her. It is only when she is certain that she is truly loved and that her lover is indeed devoted to her and will not change his mind, that she should give herself up to him. After losing her virginity she should tell her confidential friends about it and persuade him to marry her quickly.

COURTSHIP HINTS

When a girl begins to show her love by outward signs and motions, as described above, the lover should try to gain her completely by various ways and means, such as the following:

- When engaged with her in any game or sport he should intentionally hold her hand. He should find ways to lightly brush up against her.

- When engaged in water sports, he should dive at a distance from her, and come up close to her.

- He should show an increased liking for the new foliage of trees in spring and suchlike things.

- He should describe to her the pangs he suffers on her account.

- He should relate to her a beautiful dream he has had about another woman.

- At parties he should sit near her and touch her under some pretense or other, and having placed his foot upon hers, he should slowly touch each of her toes.

- Whenever he gives anything to her or takes anything from her, he should show her by his manner and look how much he loves her.

- Whenever he sits with her on the same couch he should say to her, 'I have something to tell you in private,' and then, when she comes to hear it in a quiet place, he should express his love to her more by manner and signs than by words.

Once he comes to know that she has feelings for him, he should pretend to be ill and make her come to his house. There he should intentionally hold her hand and place it on his eyes and forehead, and under the pretense of preparing some medicine for him he should ask her to do the work for his sake in the following words: 'This work must be done by you, and by nobody else.' When she wants to go away he should let her go, with an earnest request to come and see him again. This device of illness should be continued for three days and three nights. After this, when she begins coming to see him frequently, he should carry on long conversations with her, for, as the sage Ghotakamukha says, 'though a man loves a girl ever so much, he never succeeds in winning her without a great deal of talking'.

Eventually, once he knows the state of her love by all the ways she has responded at religious ceremonies, weddings, fairs, festivals, theaters, public gatherings, and like occasions, he should begin to enjoy her when she is alone, for Vatsyayana lays it down that women, when resorted to at proper times and places, do not turn away from their lovers. As for the saying that women grow less timid than usual during the evening and in darkness, and are more desirous of sex at those times, it is only talk.

Marrying for Money

A verse applies here: 'A girl who is much sought after should marry the man that she wants, one who she thinks would be obedient to her and capable of giving her pleasure. But when from the desire of wealth a girl is married by her parents to a rich man without taking into consideration the character or looks of the bridegroom, she never becomes attached to him, even though he be endowed with good qualities, obedient to her will, active, strong, healthy, and anxious to please her in every way.

A husband who is obedient but also master of himself, even if he is poor and not good-looking, is better than one who keeps company with other women, no matter how handsome and attractive he is. The wives of such men are not generally attached to their husbands; they don't confide in them, and even though they might enjoy all the external advantages of life, such wives will have recourse to lovers. Of all the lovers an unmarried girl might favor, the only one who is her true husband possesses qualities she actually likes, and such a husband alone can claim real authority over her, because he is a husband of love.

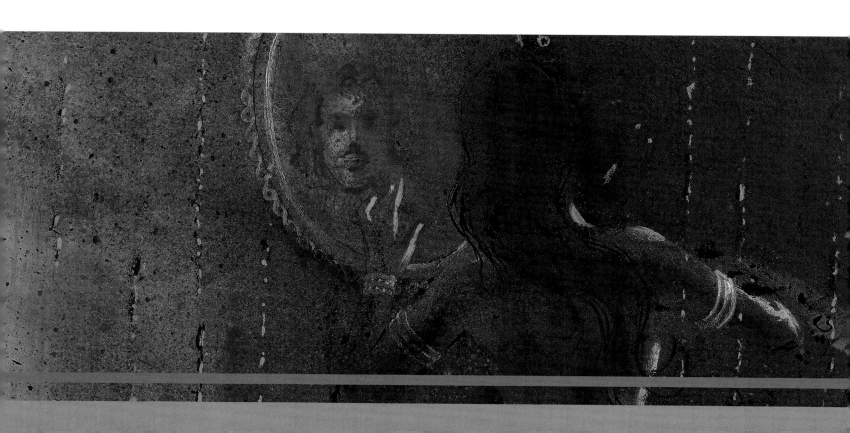

TEN DEGREES OF LOVE

The degrees of love are ten in number and are distinguished by the following marks:

- Pleasing the eyes
- Infatuated thoughts
- Constantly thinking about the loved one
- Destruction of sleep
- Emaciation of the body
- Turning away from objects of enjoyment
- Removal of shame
- Madness
- Fainting
- Death

Ancient authors declare that a man can tell from the shape and marks of a woman's body her whole disposition, truthfulness, purity, and will, not overlooking the intensity or weakness of her passions. But Vatsyayana is of the opinion that the forms of bodies, and the characteristic marks or signs, are misleading tests of character, and that women should be judged by their conduct, by the outward expression of their thoughts, and by their movements.

Now, as a general rule, Gonikaputra says that a woman falls in love with every handsome man she sees, and so does every man at the sight of a beautiful woman, but frequently they do not take any further steps, owing to various considerations.

In love the following circumstances are peculiar to the woman: She loves without regard to right or wrong, She does not try to get a man simply to carry out an ulterior purpose. When a man makes up to her she naturally shrinks from him, even though she may be willing to unite herself with him. It takes repeated and renewed entreaties before she will concede to what he wants.

But a man, even when he begins to fall in love, will conquer his feelings if morality and wisdom demand it. Even when he begins to think about the woman all the time, he doesn't yield in such circumstances, even though attempts are made to win him over. If he has made an effort to win the object of his affections, only to fail, he will stop trying and leave her alone in the future. And yet, if he does manage to win her, a man often turns indifferent to a woman. As for the opinion that a man doesn't care for what is easily gained and wants what can only be gained with great difficulty, that is so much empty talk.

WINNERS IN LOVE

The various kinds of men who generally obtain success with women are as follows:

- Men who are versed in the art and science of love
- Men who are skilled in telling stories
- Men who are acquainted with women in childhood
- Self-confident men
- Men who send presents
- Good talkers
- Men who do the things women like
- Men who haven't slept with other women yet
- Men playing the part of messengers
- Men who know their own weaknesses
- Men who are desired by good women
- Men who know a woman's friends
- Handsome, good-looking men
- Men whom a woman knows from childhood
- Neighbors
- Men devoted to sexual pleasure
- Recent bridegrooms
- Men who like parties and picnics
- Men who are liberal and generous
- 'Bull men' who are celebrated for being strong
- Enterprising and courageous men
- Men who are better-looking than a woman's husband, who exceed him in learning, generosity, and other qualities
- Men who are magnificent in their dress and lifestyle

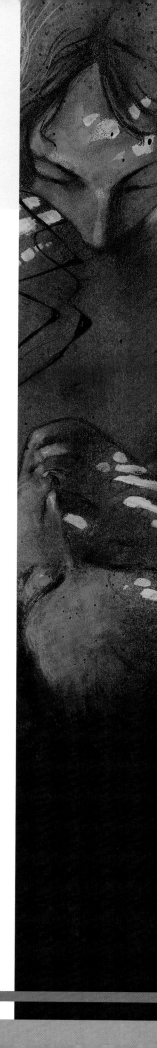

EASY WOMEN

The following kinds of women are in general easily gained over:

- Women who stand in the door of their house
- Women who are always looking out on the street
- Women who spend a lot of time at their neighbor's talking
- A woman who always stares at you
- A woman who acts as a go-between
- A woman who looks sideways at you
- Women who hate their husbands or are hated by them
- A woman who has no one to look after her and keep her in check
- Childless women
- A woman whose child has died
- Social butterflies and party girls
- A woman who acts overaffectionately with her husband
- An actor's wife
- Widows
- Poor women
- A woman who likes to enjoy herself
- The wife of a man who has many younger brothers
- Vain women
- A woman whose husband is inferior to her in ability

- A woman who is proud of her artistic achievements
- A woman who is disturbed because her husband has cheated on her
- A woman who married a rich man when she was too young and now desires someone closer to her own tastes
- Women whom their husbands have slighted without cause
- A woman who is considered inferior by other women of her station
- A woman whose husband travels
- A jeweler's wife
- Jealous women
- Covetous women
- Immoral women
- Barren women
- Lazy women
- Cowardly women
- A humpback
- A dwarf
- Deformed women
- Loud and vulgar women
- Women who smell bad
- A sick woman
- Older women

ADVICE FOR SEDUCERS

Some ancient authors hold that girls are not so easily seduced by employing female go-betweens as by the efforts of the man himself; however, the wives of others are more easily got at by the aid of go-betweens than by the personal efforts of the man. Vatsyayana lays it down that whenever it is possible a man should always act for himself in these matters, and it is only when this is impracticable or impossible that female go-betweens should be employed. As for the saying that women who act and talk boldly and freely are to be won by the personal efforts of the man, and that women who do not possess these qualities are to be got at by go-betweens, it is only a matter of talk.

When a man is trying to seduce one woman he should not attempt to seduce any other at the same time. But after he has succeeded with the first and enjoyed her for a considerable time, he can keep her affections by giving her presents and then commence making up to another woman. When a man sees the husband of a woman going somewhere near home, he should not enjoy the woman then, even though she may be easily gained over at that time. A wise man having a regard for his reputation should not think of seducing a woman who is apprehensive, timid, not to be trusted, well guarded, or possessed of a father-in-law or mother-in-law.

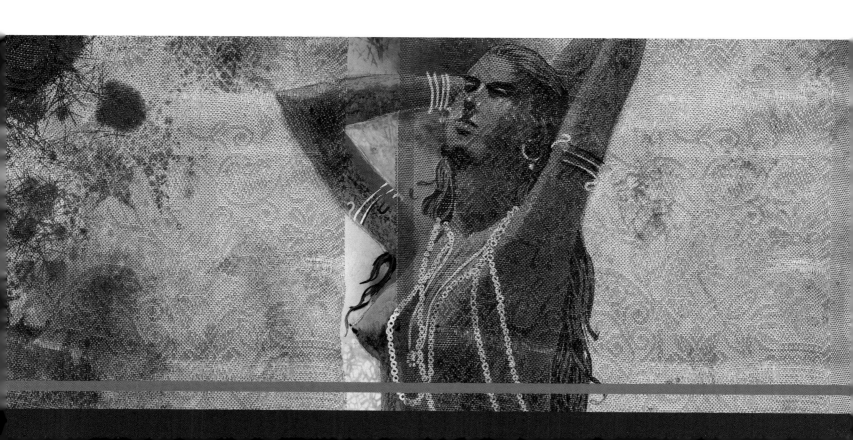

READING A WOMAN'S MIND

When a man is trying to gain over a woman he should try to read her mind and act as follows: if she listens to him but doesn't show in any way her own intentions, he should try to gain her over by means of a go-between. If she meets him once and comes to meet him a second time better dressed than before, or if she meets him in some lonely place, he can be certain that she is capable of being enjoyed with the use of a little force. A woman who lets a man make up to her but doesn't give herself to him, even after a long time, should be considered as a tease, a trifler in love; owing to the fickleness of the human mind, however, even such a woman can be conquered by always keeping up a close acquaintance with her.

When a woman avoids the attentions of a man and on account of respect for him, and pride in herself, will not meet him or approach him, she can be gained over with difficulty, either by trying to keep on familiar terms with her or by an exceedingly clever go-between.

When a man makes up to a woman and she reproaches him with harsh words, she should be abandoned at once. But when a woman reproaches a man and at the same time acts affectionately toward him, she should be made love to in every way.

A woman who meets a man in lonely places and puts up with the touch of his foot but pretends, on account of the indecision of her mind, not to be aware of it, should be conquered by patience and continued efforts as follows: if she happens to go to sleep in his vicinity he should put his left arm around her and see when she awakes whether she has been repulsing him for real or only in such a way as if she wanted the same thing done to her again. And what is done by the arm can also be done by the foot. If the man succeeds up to this point he should embrace her more closely. If she pushes him away and gets up, but behaves with him as usual the next day, he should consider that she is not unwilling to be enjoyed by him. If, however, she does not appear again, the man should try to get over her by means of a go-between; and if, after having disappeared for some time, she again appears and behaves with him as usual, the man should then consider that she would not object to having sex with him.

When a woman gives a man an opportunity and makes her love manifest to him, he should proceed to enjoy her. The signs of a woman manifesting her love are these:

- She calls out to a man without being addressed by him first
- She shows herself to him in secret places
- She speaks to him inarticulately or with trembling voice
- Her hands or feet are moist with perspiration, and her face is flushed with delight
- She remains with both hands placed on his body motionless as if she had been surprised by something, or was overcome by fatigue
- She places one of her hands quite motionless on his body, and even though the man should press it close, she does not remove it for a long time

Thus ends the examination of the state of a woman's mind.

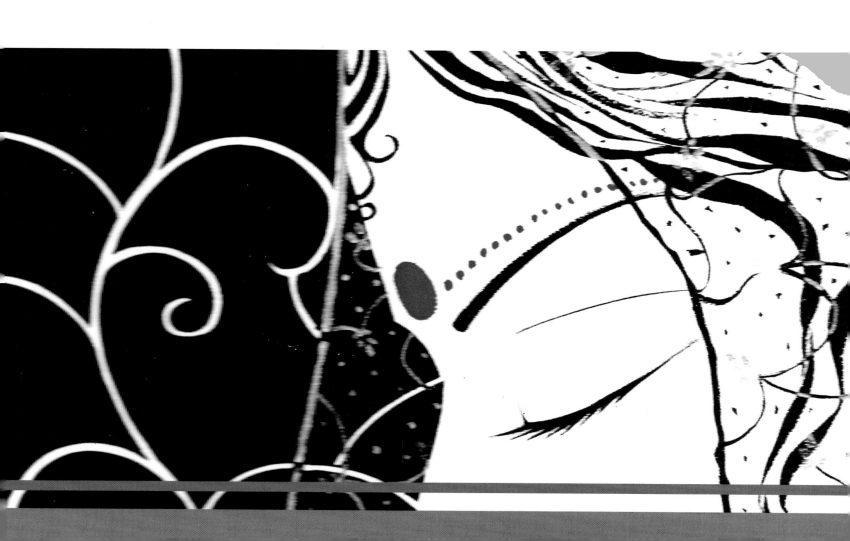

IN CONCLUSION

Thus have I written in brief the science of love, after reading the texts of ancient authors and following the ways of enjoyment taught by them. One who is acquainted with the true principles of this science pays regard to virtue (Dharma), material success (Artha), and love or pleasure (Kama), as well as to one's own experiences. Such a one is not driven simply by his own desires.

A sexual practice is not right just because it is authorized by the science; keep in mind that these rules are only to be acted upon in the right context. After reading and considering the ancient authors, and thinking over the meaning of the rules given by them, the *Kama Sutra* was composed according to the precepts of Holy Writ, for the benefit of the world, by Vatsyayana, leading the life of a religious student and wholly engaged in the contemplation of God.

This work is not intended to be used merely as an instrument for satisfying our desires. A person acquainted with the true principles of this science, and who preserves his Dharma, Artha, and Kama, and has regard for the practices of society, is sure to obtain mastery over his senses. In short, through seeking the three goals of life an intelligent and prudent person, without becoming the slave of his passions, obtains success in everything that he may undertake.

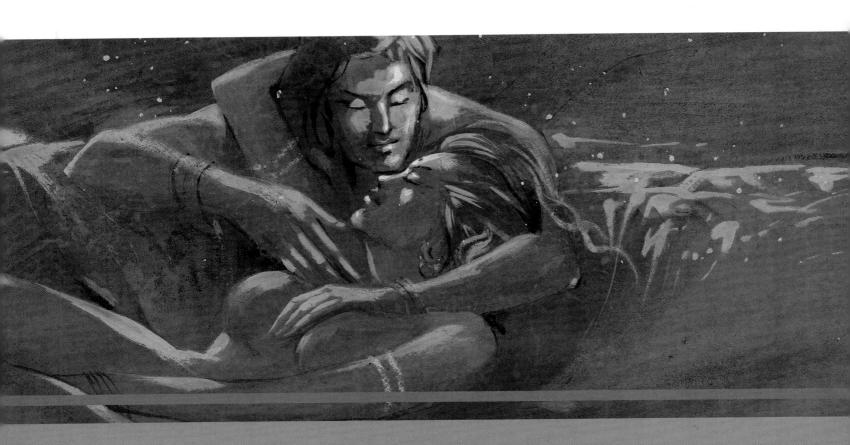

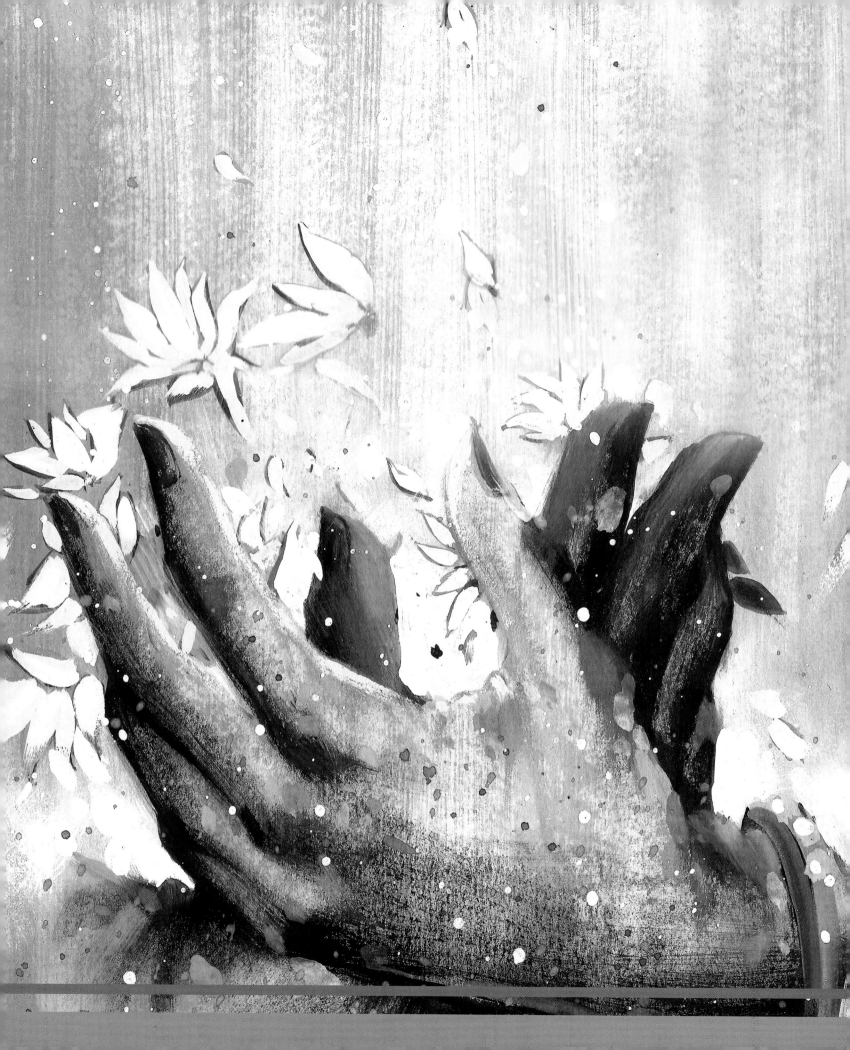

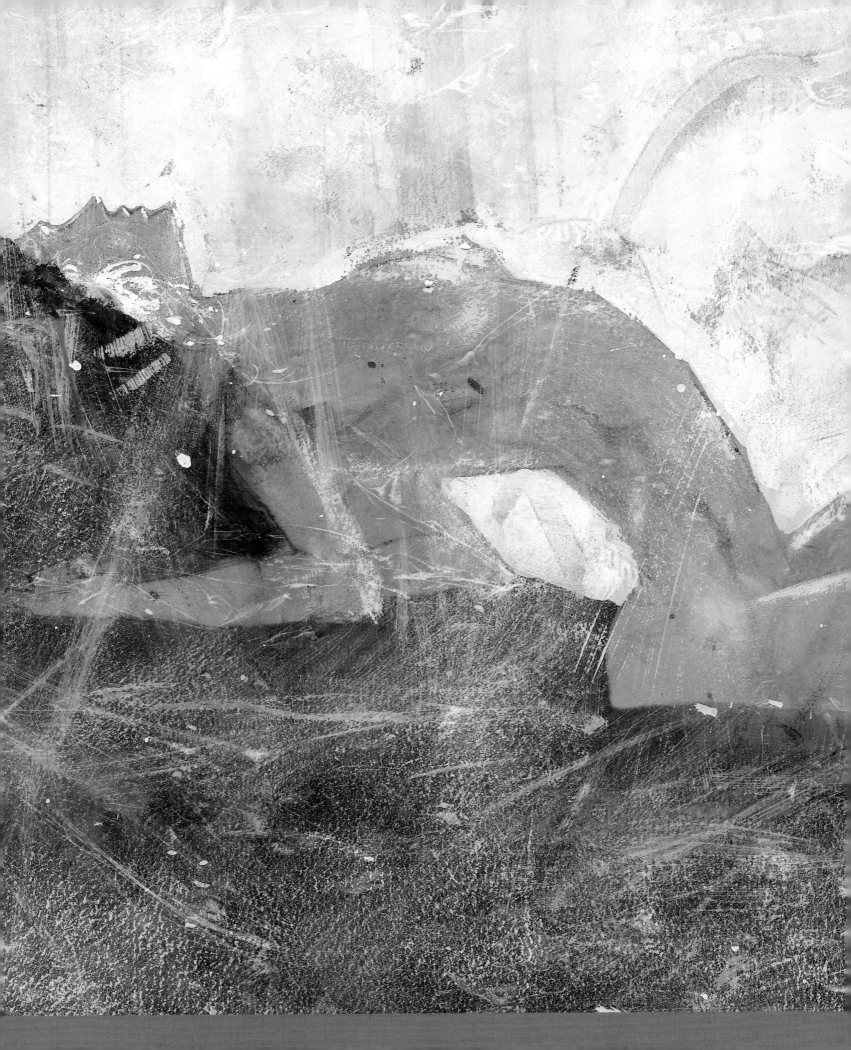

CHAPTER 3

IMAGES OF LOVE

The universe contains three things that cannot be destroyed: Being, Awareness, and Love.

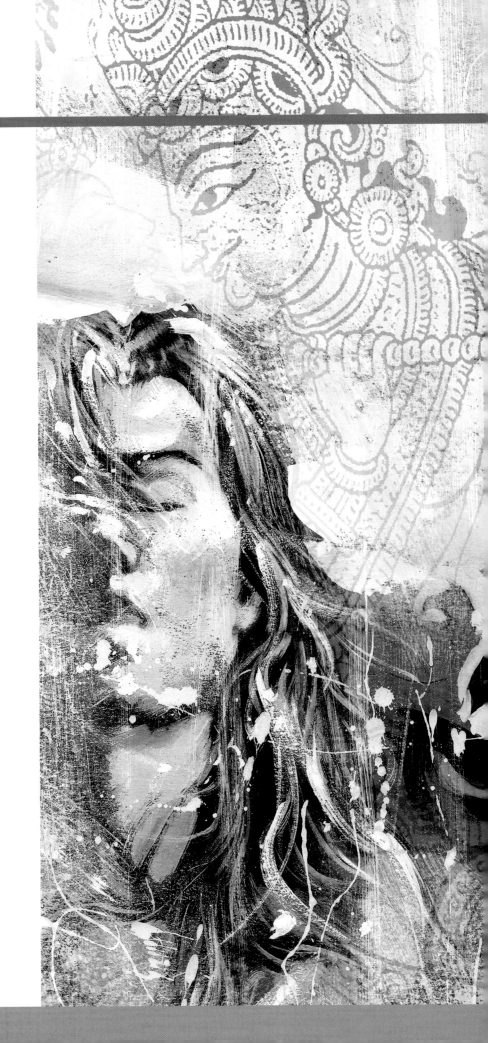

To know
what love
really is,
you must
discover
that you
are love.

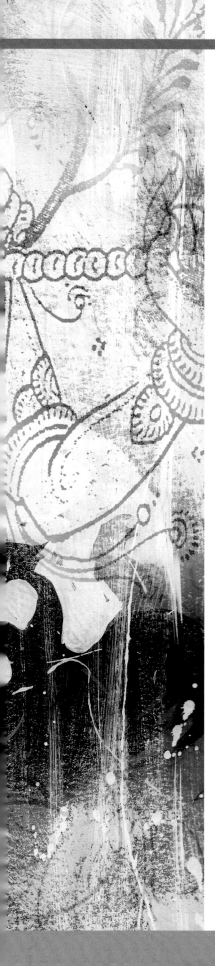

The force that makes life expand
is desire.

When a desire follows the flow of
love, it benefits all of life.

When desire is blocked, growth
cannot happen naturally.

What does it mean to grow?
It means letting life be new at
any moment.

Desire is the heart's way
of reaching into the
unknown.

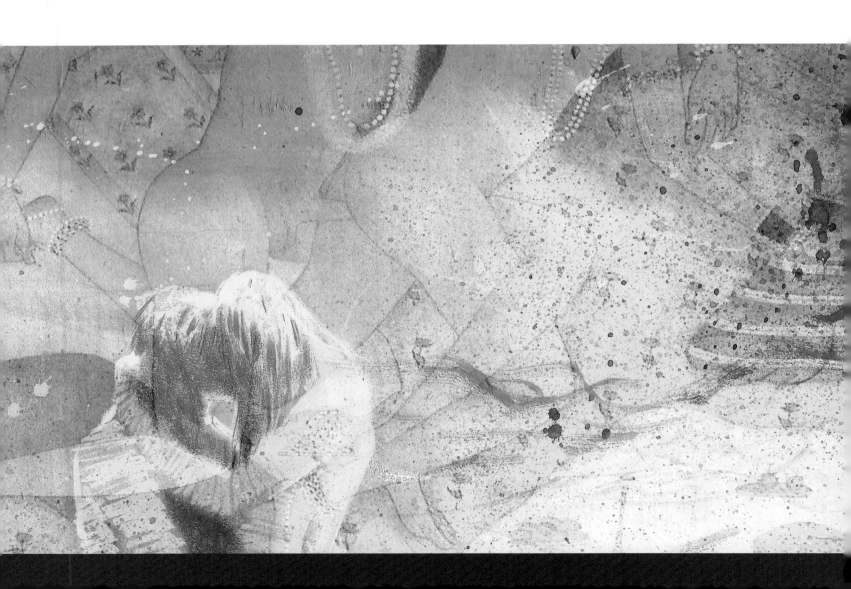

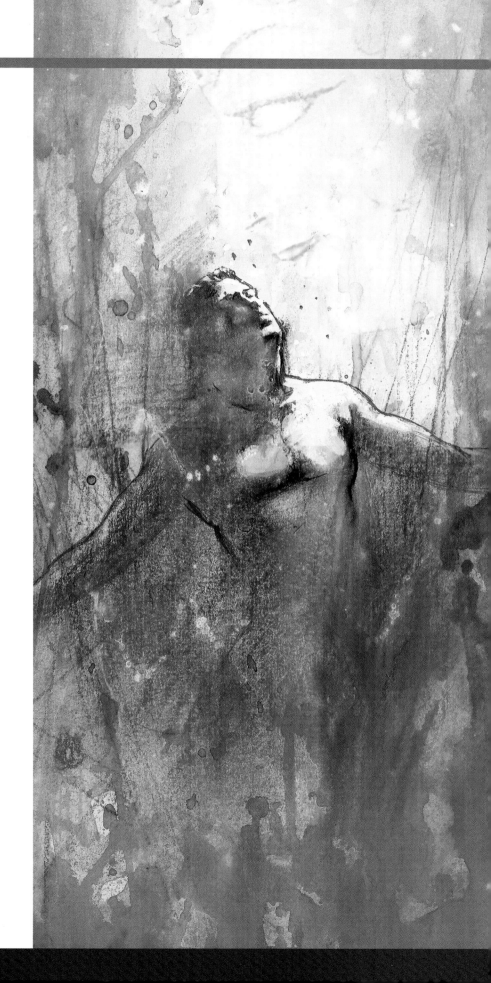

Losing yourself in sex is a pleasure. Finding yourself in sex is a blessing.

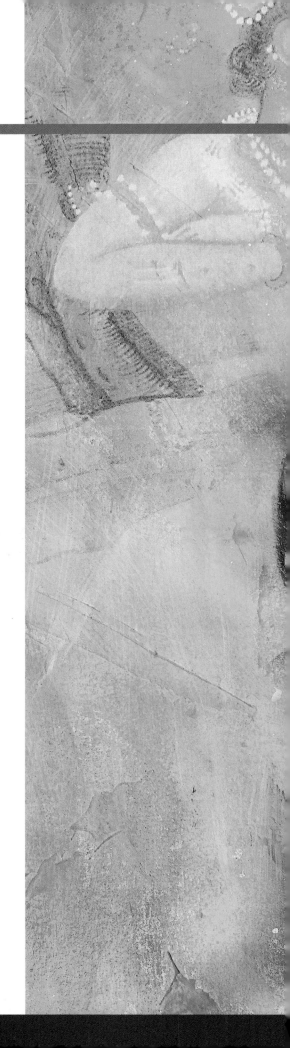

When you can cherish the
unknown — in yourself and in
others — you have become
a lover.

For everyone love is the journey.
Those we call lovers realize that
this is true.

Love is constant. The journey is
our way of experiencing an
illusion: that love can change.

Love is everywhere and nowhere
at the same time — like Being.
Like God.

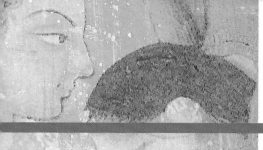

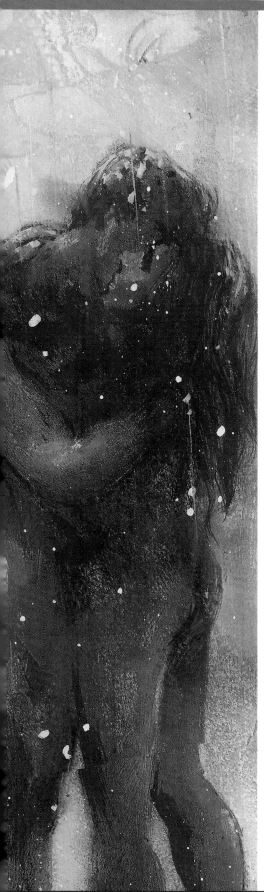

Today your love depends on how you feel and act. Tomorrow, if you are fortunate, it will depend on nothing.

When love comes, it feels as if it has found you. In truth you remembered to look for it.

97

Love isn't fickle. It only comes and goes because we do.

Universal love is the expansion of personal love. Personal love is the concentration of universal love.

Loving someone else is
the same as loving God.
One person is a wave;
God is the whole ocean.

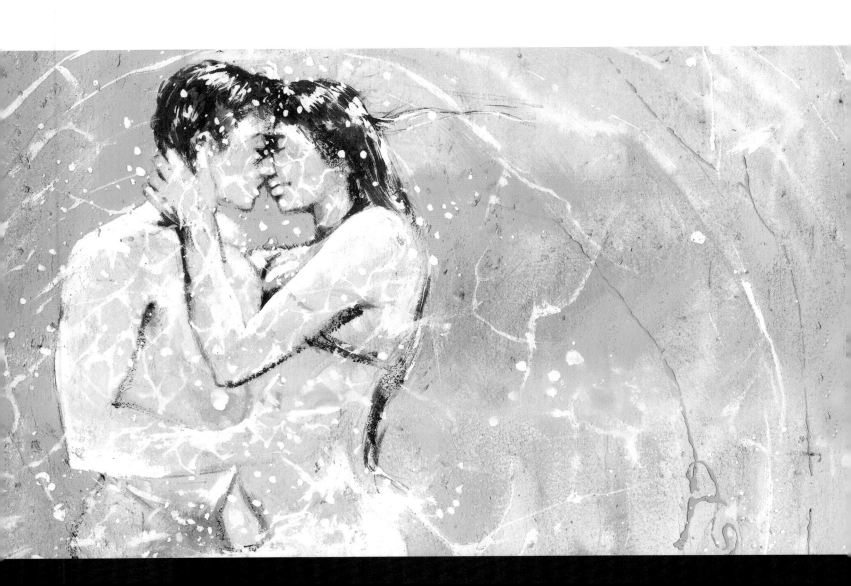

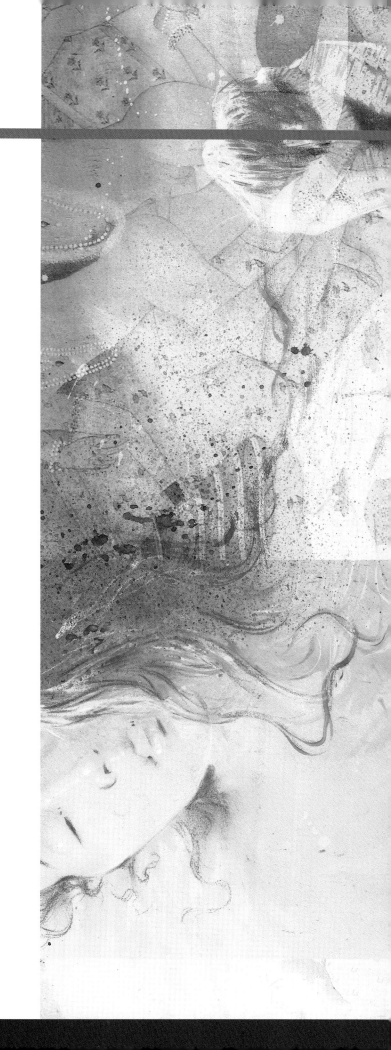

Life is one flow of love, which the mind separates into good and bad. In that separation it creates good and bad.

The love you pray for is trying to reach you at every moment.
So pray for the highest love. Then when it reaches you, your blessing will be infinite.

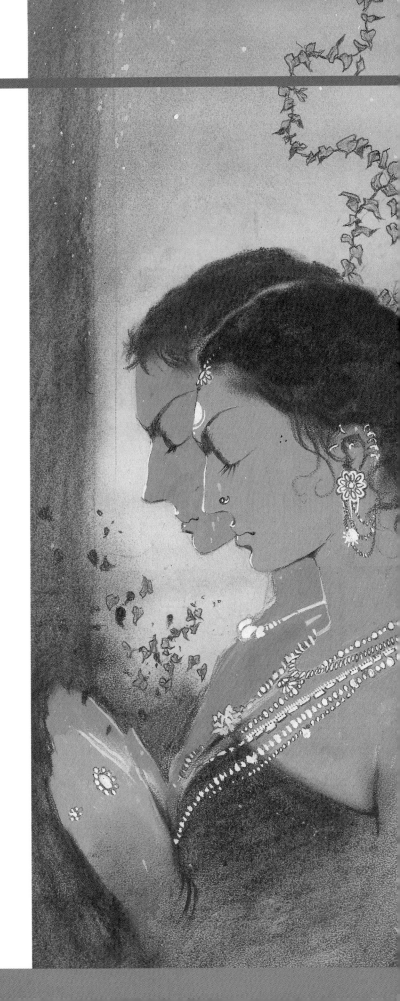

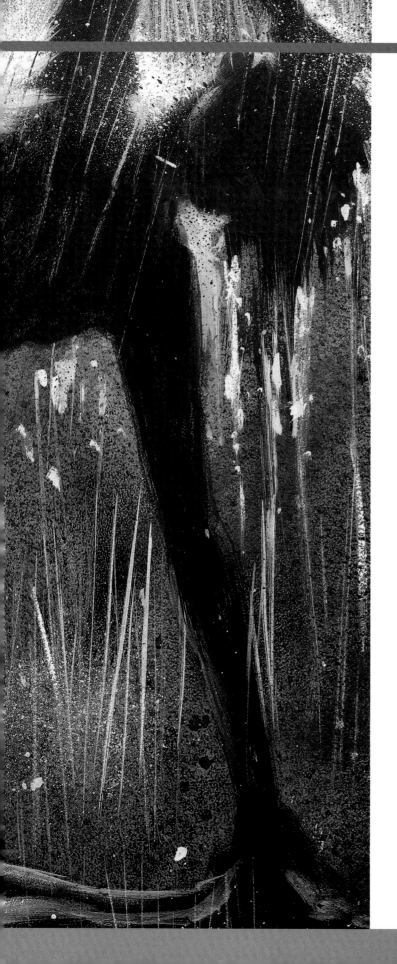

Purity is the secret of fulfilling your desires. The purest heart brings the highest love.

All prayers ask for love, no matter what they seem to be asking for. Healing is love, a deep wish is love, God's attention is love.

Lovers seem to fly to an unreal world. Actually they are the only ones who can make this world real.

Desires come true when they are held quietly in the heart.

Don't shout your dreams to the world — whisper them to love.

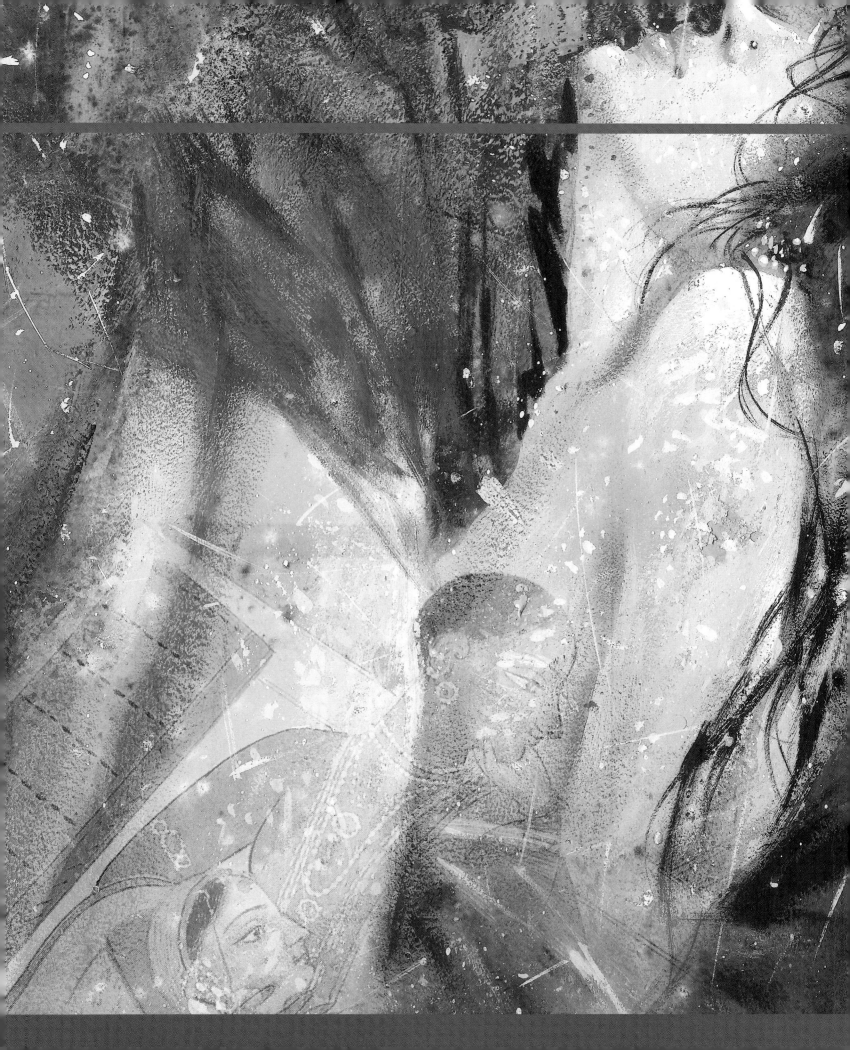

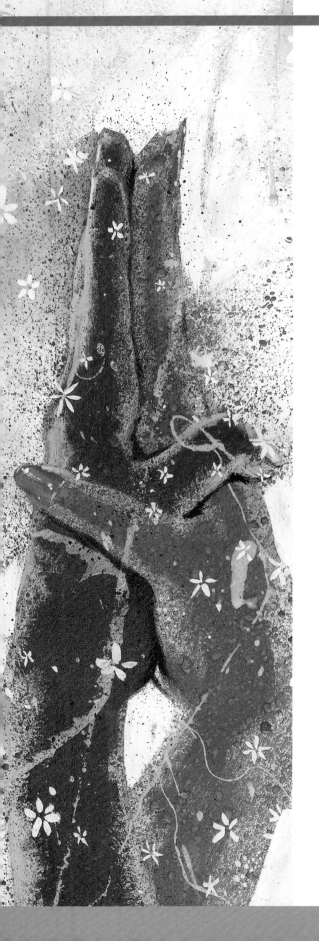

When lovers meet, one part of God is taking pleasure in another part of God.

If making love feels like being a god, remember that the gods invented it.

What's the universe doing right now? It's eavesdropping on your every desire.

Even those who hunger for pleasures of the flesh are actually seeking the soul in disguise.

What does not contain love must contain an illusion.

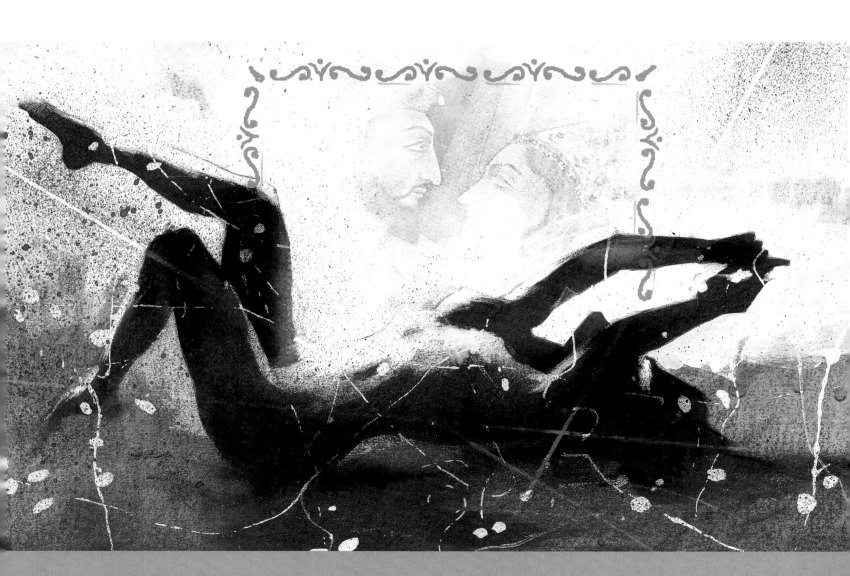

Every desire, even those you judge
against, is trying to heal your
lack of love.

When you ask, 'Who am I?' the right
answer is, 'I am love.' Every other
answer is an illusion that will eventually
pass away.

In love all things are made new.

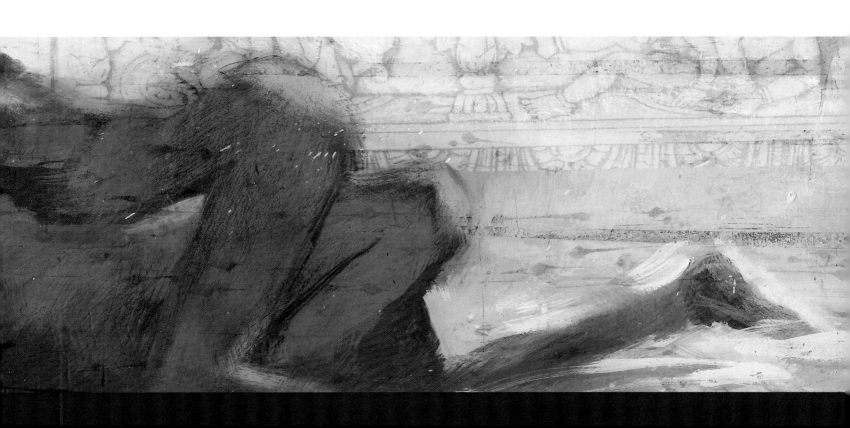

Pleasure is the smile that love bestows
on mortality.

Death is an illusion. The closest it comes
to being real is when love is absent.

The beauty you see in life is a reflection
of the beauty you see in yourself.
The love you feel in life is a reflection
of the love you feel in yourself.

107

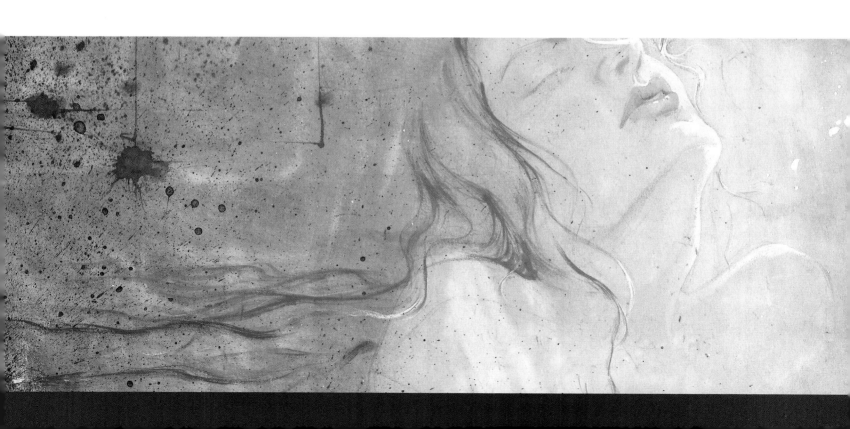

108

Sex is a paradox.
It needs the
difference between
man and woman,
yet it reminds them
that they are not
different at all.
In this way pleasure
is the world's great
equalizer.

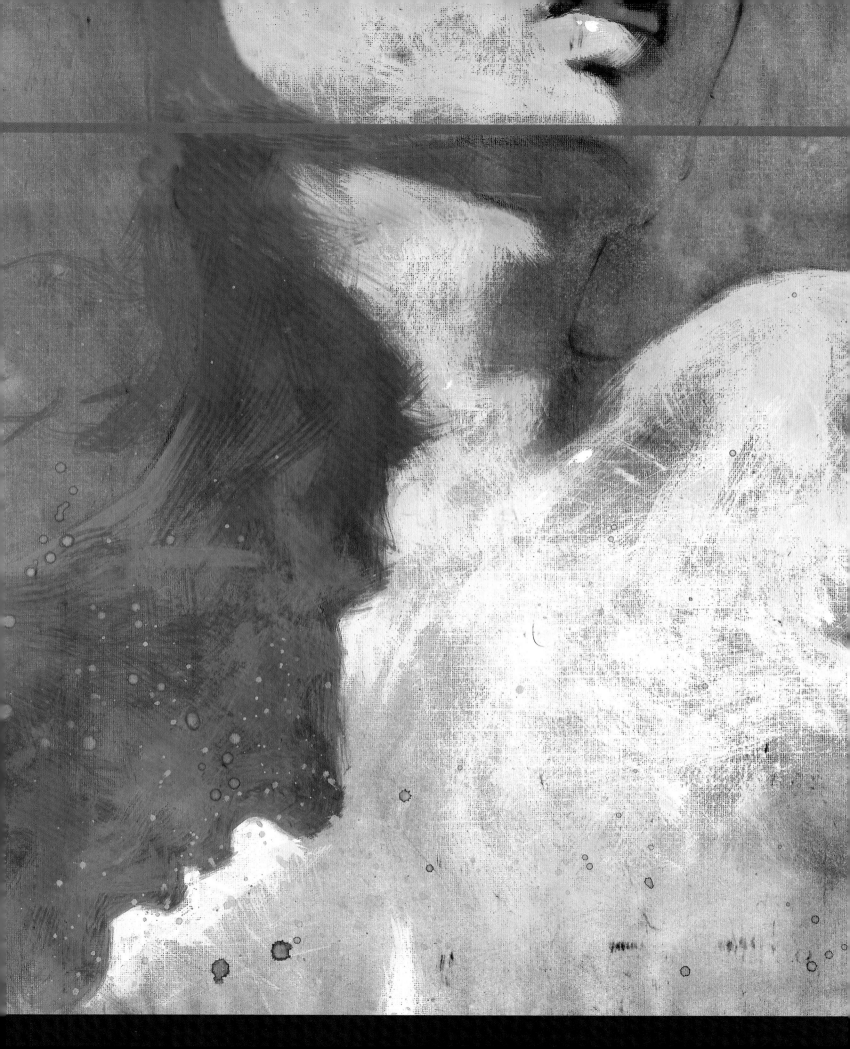

If you want to decode human nature, look closely at those who love and those who don't. In love's crucible there are no secrets.

The mystery of love is that nothing is more selfish, and yet nothing so purifies selfishness away.

You want to know if you grew today? Then ask if you loved something new today.

In sex we reveal who we are. Lovers rejoice in this; those who only pretend to love hate it.

Sex is nourishing, but sex without love is like trying to grow a rose with sun but no water.

The union which pleases God most isn't the union of man and woman. It is the union of sex and love.

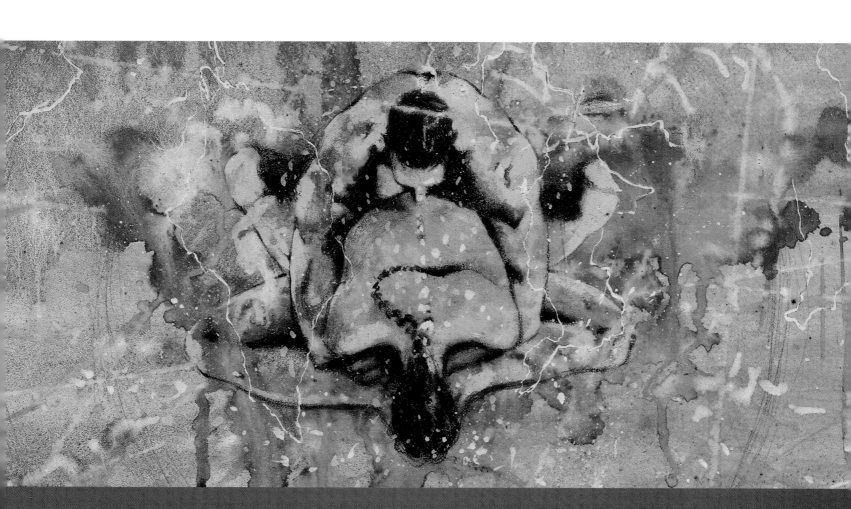

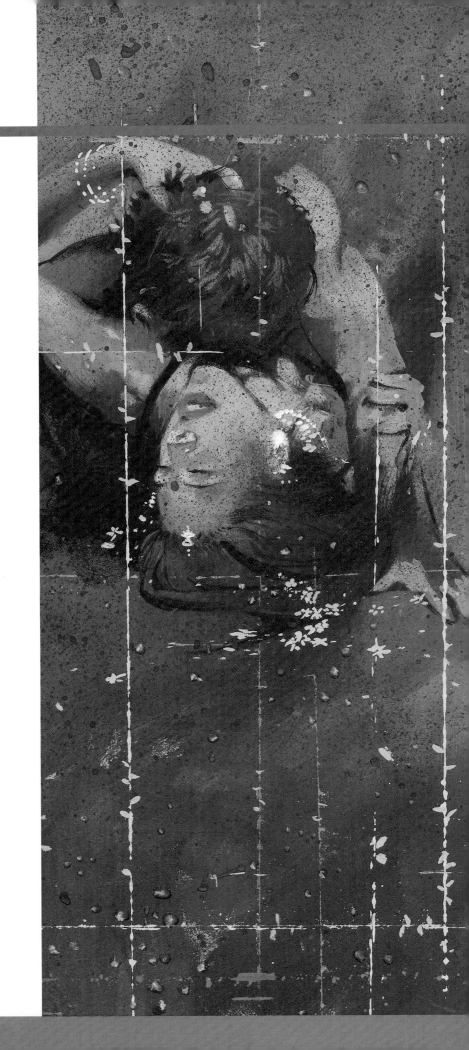

Sex isn't the
original sin.
Guilt is.

Orgasm is that fleeting moment when
the burden of the self is gone.

Orgasm is the body's bliss. If you add
love, it becomes the soul's bliss.

To please a woman is to please a goddess.
To please a man is to please a god.

The greatest pleasure one can
experience is just a hint of the soul's
possibilities.

Sex and bliss are related as a single rose
is related to the garden of Paradise.

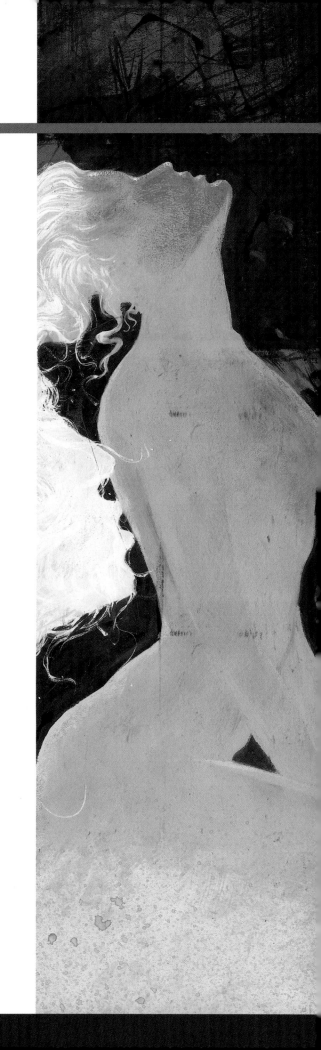

Ask me what pleasure is and
I will know you've never
experienced it. Pleasure
needs no words unless it is
absent. The same is true of
happiness, and love itself.

What is truth?
Love in action.

When making love, a lover
gives all gifts and asks
for none.

The madness of lovers makes
sanity seem like so much dust
in the wind.

Innocence is the ability
to give and receive love
without holding on.

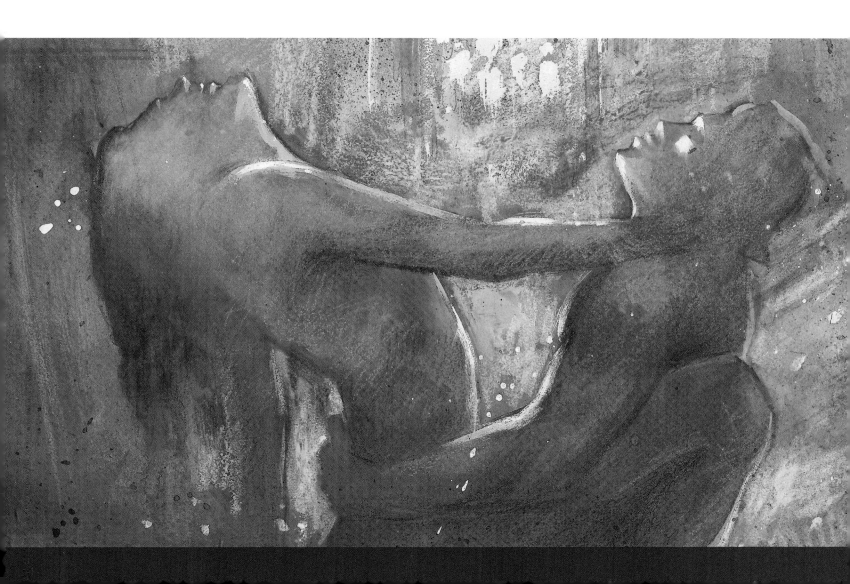

Sex wasn't God's big mistake. Judging against sex was humanity's big mistake. Pleasure is as divine as any cathedral, any temple.

115

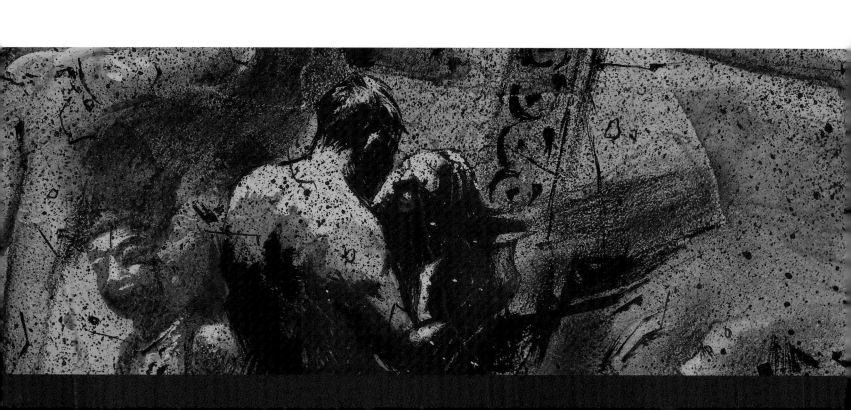

Spirit and flesh have never been
separate. They keep apart just to flirt.

All wrongs in the world arise from a
belief in non-love.

You want a scripture you can believe in?
Read your lover's eyes.

117

Don't yearn for some faraway heaven.
This world plus love is heaven.

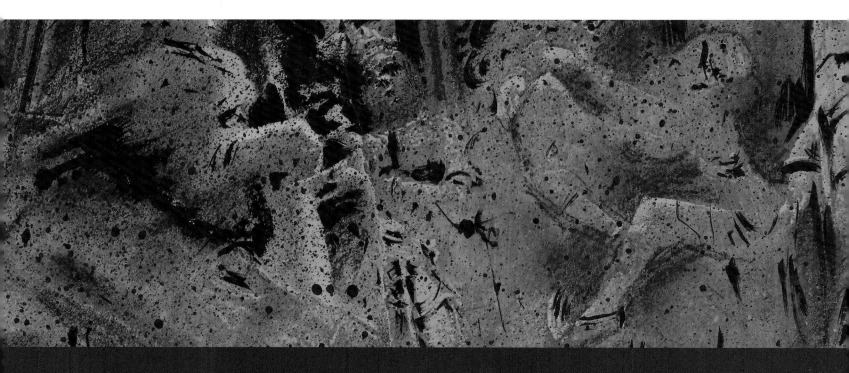

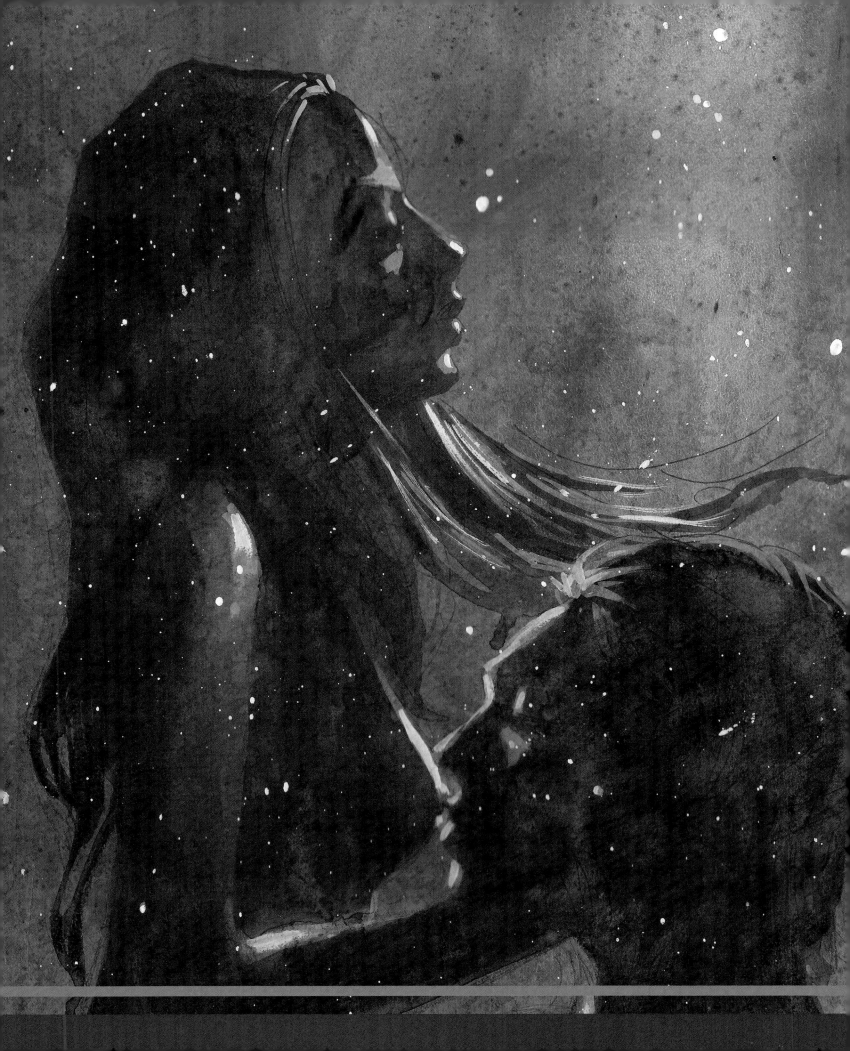

CHAPTER 4

UNITING SEX AND LOVE

It seems almost miraculous that the Kama Sutra still speaks to us, and it gives great pleasure to celebrate that fact. But values change as societies do, and 'the art of love' is no exception.

The Kama Sutra comes down to us from a society dominated by priests and temples. Its advice, therefore, is much more sexually free than spiritually so. There was little room for husband and wife to find a spiritual path for themselves through sex. They were expected to make love without shame and with pleasure in mind; the deeper union of sex and spirit is unspoken in Vatsyayana's world (his truly spiritual lovers are all gods and goddesses).

I couldn't leave the *Kama Sutra* without expanding on this topic, because in our time sex is talked about incessantly, with very confused results. In my experience what couples want is a way out of this confusion. Having tried sex much earlier and more freely than any previous generation, they are not frightened by it — rather, they wonder what it really means. After your thousandth orgasm, is sex as worn out as anything else? Why hasn't it revealed the hidden glory of another person, or of yourself?

A hundred years ago, when repression was respectable, an ideal form of love was supposed to bind men and women. Married love was blessed as long as it had no genitals. The eminent Victorian writer John Ruskin, who learned about female anatomy from Greek statues, ran from the bridal chamber in horror when he discovered on his honeymoon that his wife had pubic hair. Sweaty, undignified sex was not accepted as an aspect of ideal love; in the guise of carnal lust, sex all but killed idealism. Didn't they hear Shakespeare himself lamenting sex as 'The expense of spirit in a waste of shame'?

This ugly belief system persists today in different circles. Fundamentalist Christians who are convinced that sex repeats original sin would be surprised to find themselves in agreement with New Age followers of Eastern religion for whom purity and celibacy are also the ideal way to approach sex. Avoid it if you can, indulge if you must. Turn away in disgust at the very thought of promiscuity and homosexuality. Anyone who believes naively that Eastern religions are more tolerant of either will be rudely awakened when they ask an orthodox Buddhist or Hindu for advice. I vividly recall a prominent Ayurvedic physician who had traveled to America in the mid-80s to extol the healing benefits of traditional Indian medicine. At a press conference a reporter asked him about what Ayurveda could do for AIDS. A look of horror crossed the venerable doctor's face. 'AIDS? One man, one woman. That is God's law,' he intoned.

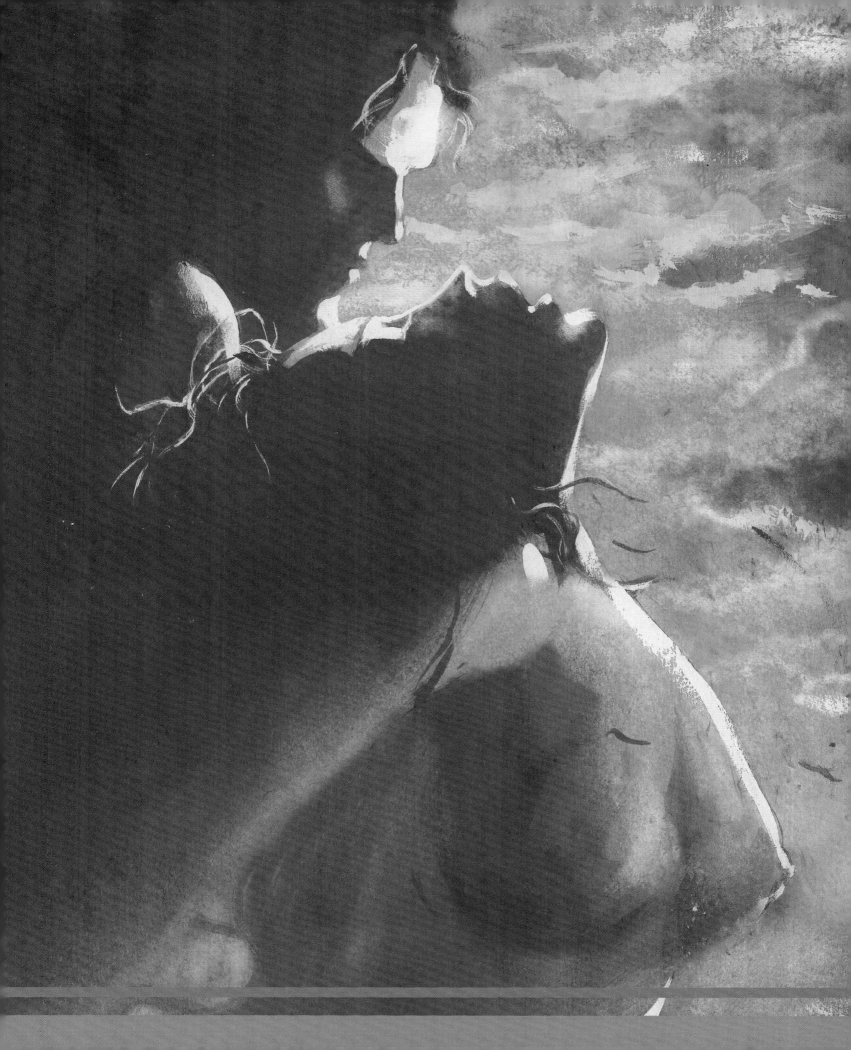

But ours is a society of free choice, and in secular circles sex is openly discussed and accepted. Here, the great bugaboo is disease, for when sin went out the window, the specter of STDs came in, and today's schoolchildren are hit with horror stories of what can happen if they take even a single sexual misstep. Love your partner but be careful he (or she) doesn't destroy your life. Almost the only echo of the *Kama Sutra*'s sane regard for pleasure comes in men's magazines, where the fantasy side of sex is indulged in completely — and we must nod toward the feminist movement for allowing women's magazines their own brand of runaway fantasy.

How can we begin to think of sex as a spiritual force? Although he didn't go far enough, Vatsyayana did think of it that way. But to be frank, he also understood how seemingly destructive the sexual urge can be. After thousands of years, sex remains frightening in its power to totally strip a person of common sense, self-control, moderation, dignity, peacefulness, and sleep. Sexual fantasies roam the mind at will. We have little control over them, and when they touch our dark places of shame and guilt, what begins in physical pleasure can turn into suffering and obsession.

I think the *Kama Sutra* shows a way out of this dark maze — or at least it points the way. We haven't freed ourselves by becoming sexually more explicit, anymore than we became free of crime by showing every lurid murder on television. There is a secret here, and the secret is that sex is freedom. It has that in common with love. One cannot claim that sex and love are automatically the same, because millions of sex acts (and fantasies) are performed out of sheer selfishness, without the slightest hint of love. But sex brings freedom by the very way it strips us down, makes us free of ego, renders dignity and self-control ridiculous. When sex is actually united with love, its ability to free someone becomes amazingly strong. No wonder that in every civilization the gods and goddesses of love also joined their bodies in sex.

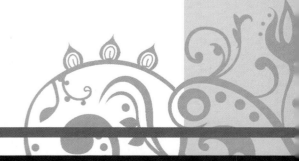

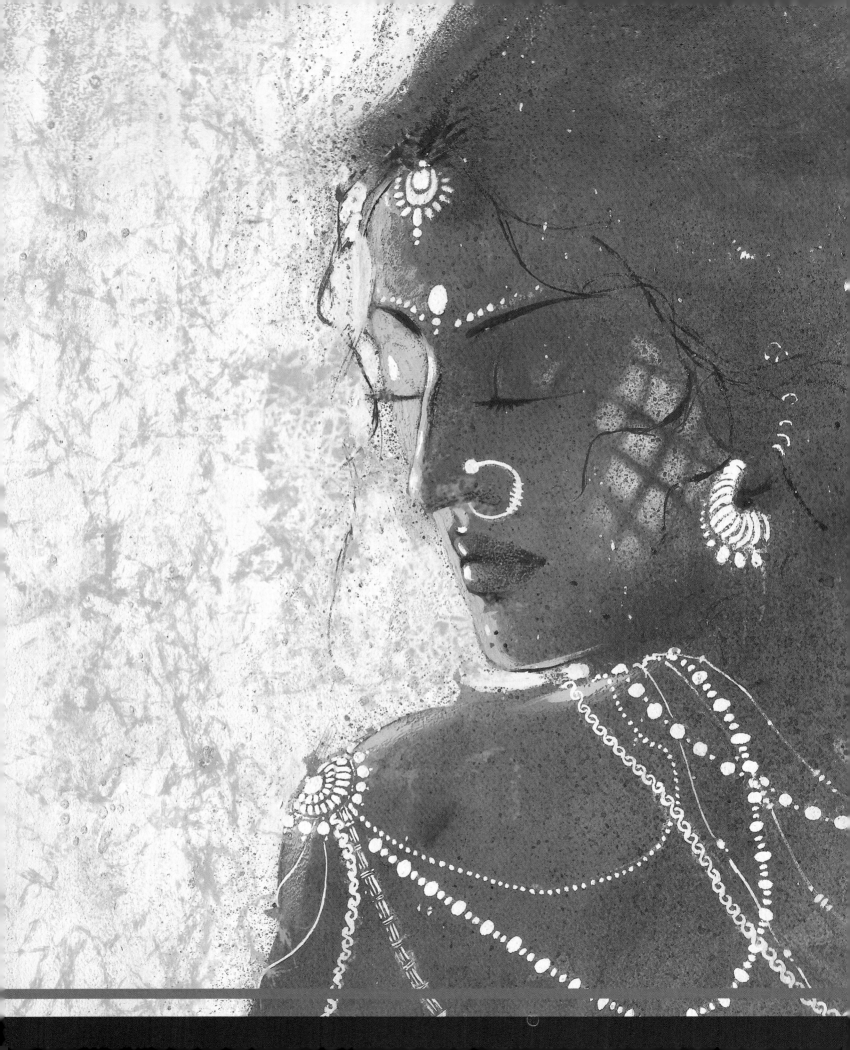

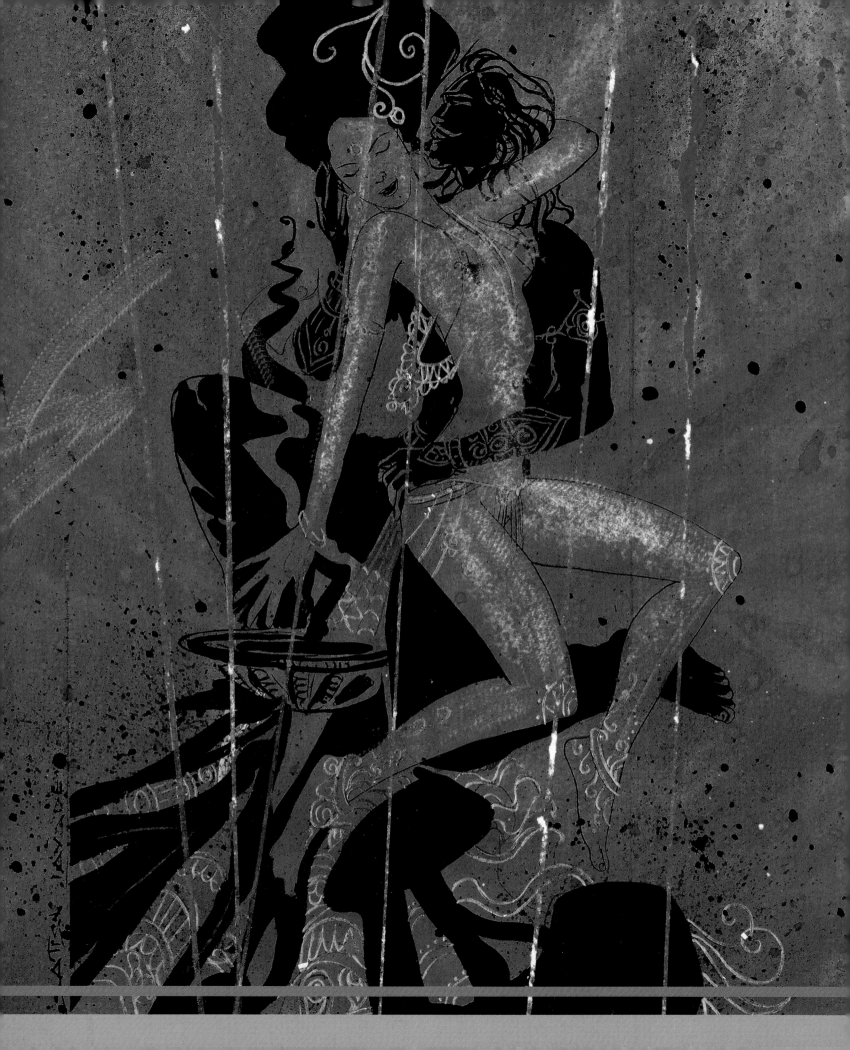

THE EXPERIENCE OF ECSTASY

Sex is the main way that billions of people experience ecstasy, and ecstasy is a spiritual value poised precariously in the realm of the physical.

You split me, and tore my heart open. You filled me with love. You poured your spirit into mine. I knew you as I know myself. My eyes are radiant with your light. My ears delight in your music. My nostrils are filled with your fragrance. My face is covered with your dew. You have made all things new. You have made me see all things shining. You have granted me perfect ease. I have become like Paradise.

This uninhibited proclamation of ecstasy is very old. The words are part of a collection of verses in the ancient language of Syriac discovered in 1909. Biblical scholars believe that the original text was probably written before the first century AD, and call them the Odes of Solomon. They express the ravishing ecstasy of love at its most intense. Ecstasy is a primordial energy state, and love is meant to take us there. Ecstasy is also where we come from. The pre-eminent Vedic texts of India, the *Upanishads*, declare, 'In bliss and love these creatures are born. In bliss and love, they are sustained. To bliss they return.' All yearning, all striving, all the things that we do with our lives have ecstatic love as the ultimate goal. Which implies that for a deeply spiritual person, turning one's back on sex is much the same as turning one's back on the very nature of the soul. I remember a Nobel laureate saying wistfully, 'This is a consolation prize for love. All I wanted in my whole life was love. All our exploring is really a seeking of love.'

Love is the beginning. It is also the ending. T.S. Eliot wrote, 'We shall not cease from exploration. And the end of our exploring is to arrive where we started from and know the place for the first time.' We do not have to exclude science from this loving exploration. Years ago, when I was doing my residency in internal medicine, I became aware of the healing power of love. Seriously ill patients who felt they were loved sometimes recovered against all the odds. Others with mild illnesses, who felt alone and unloved, languished and withered away into death and oblivion. Later, as the whole field of mind—body medicine burgeoned, numerous studies confirmed this, primarily by showing that when a person feels loved, the immune system is activated, along with beneficial neurotransmitters in the brain, such as dopamine and serotonin.

But how many people realize that every single beneficial chemical response in the body is triggered by sex? No other behavior can make that claim. Even the hormone associated with breast-feeding, which gives new mothers a contented glow, is also activated during sexual union. The immune system is strengthened, and so are feelings of power, peace, contentment, and belonging. In an earlier age no one linked this to biochemistry, yet with physiological proof in hand, we can banish repression as unhealthy in every way, including the physical. Be ecstatic and be well.

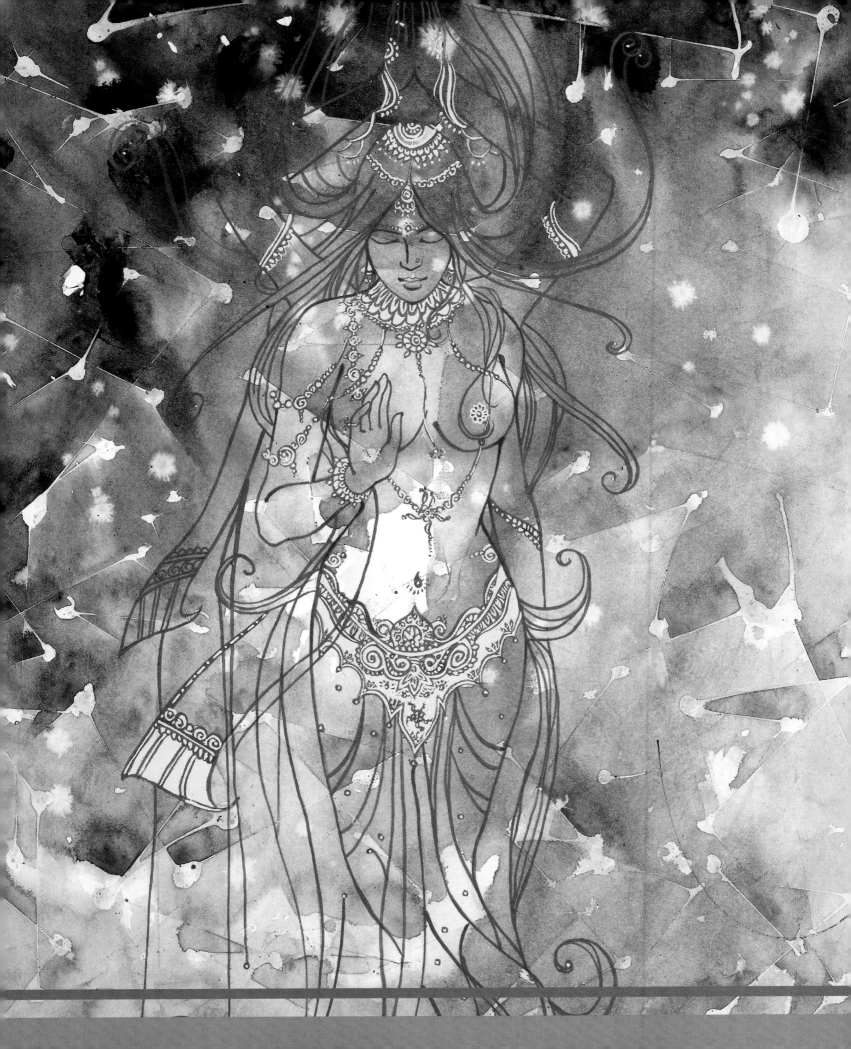

THE SEVEN STAGES
OF LOVE

The next step is a short one — if sex and wellbeing are already intimate, then sex and spirit cannot be far apart. The wisdom traditions of the world, both East and West, tell us that love, in its essence, is the force of spirit, that all love ultimately is the play of the divine. Within every love story hides the wooing of the gods and goddesses. This is one area of life where the practical meets the mythical. For many people the experience of romantic love is their first experience of spirituality, although they may not know it. All love is based on the search for spirit, and the agony of yearning is just a mask for the ecstasy of bliss. Romantic lovers experience the wisdom of uncertainty. They are full of wonder. They are exposed. They feel renewed and transformed. They become detached from the trivial and the mundane. They are spontaneous. They are vulnerable, and they are carefree. These are all spiritual qualities. If we could maintain them, we would be on our way to liberation.

How do we maintain them? By expecting to. Only if you expect romance to blossom into its full spiritual potential will it do so; otherwise, when nothing is expected of it except to stay the same, romance withers away. Nothing this powerful can stay the same, yet when falling in love disappears we blame its fickleness instead of ourselves. Only in your awareness can love grow. There is no other place, no exotic land where love flourishes like a wild orchid in the Garden of Eden. I am personally certain that man is not a fallen creature; but we are forgetful. Fortunately, the same consciousness that went to sleep can be reawakened; the real art of love, which the *Kama Sutra* only hints at, restores love to its rightful position as the seat of the soul.

If you expect love to unfold until it reaches its highest goal of ecstasy and liberation, it's necessary to understand the stages of love. There are seven of them, and they play out in physical form seven spiritual laws of love. The two go hand in hand, because it takes action before any spiritual law can be experienced; they do not exist in a vacuum. The Seven Stages of Love apply to all kinds of love: love for one's work as a scientist or artist, love for our family and children, and love for the divine, or God. If we understand the dynamics of love as it goes through these seven stages and obey the Seven Spiritual Laws, we will be able to create the love that we want in all areas of our life. Love will follow us wherever we go. We will never be able to escape it.

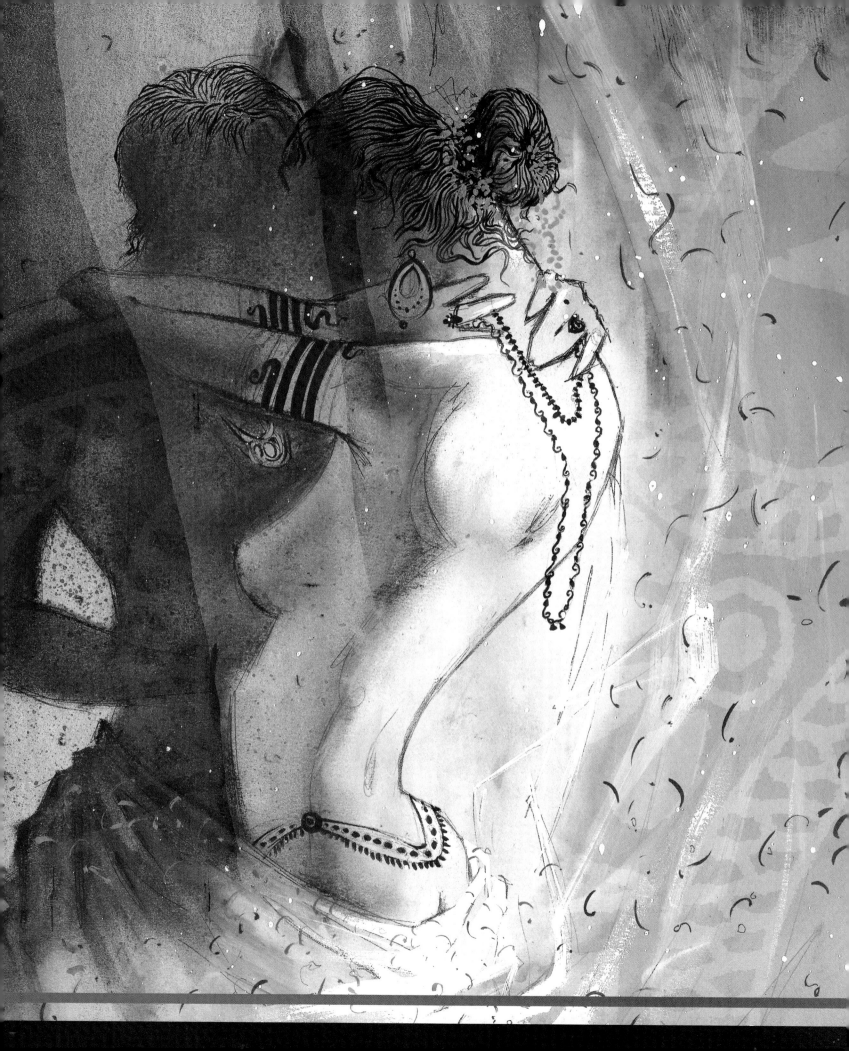

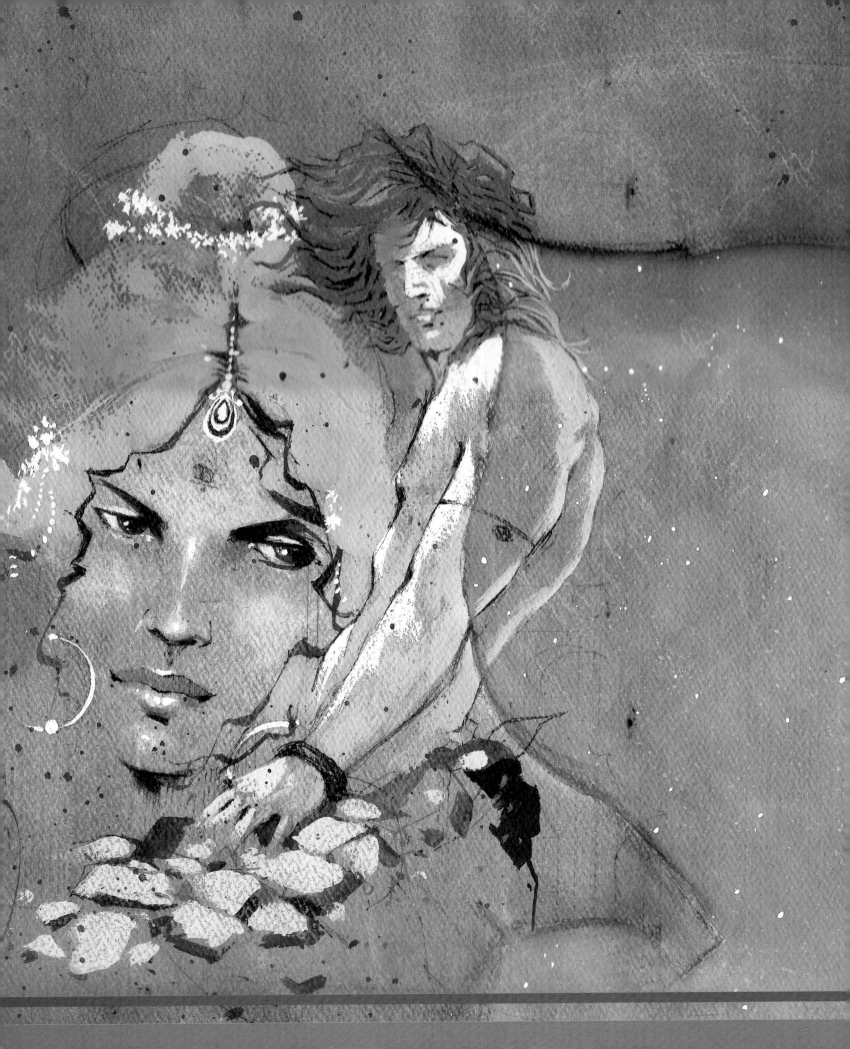

The First Stage of Love: Attraction

The Law of Attraction states, 'To be attractive, you have to be authentic.' What makes a person attractive? The wisdom traditions tell us that attraction first and foremost comes from naturalness. Nothing is more beautiful than naturalness. It alone contains the mystery and allure that spark romance. Being natural also means being comfortable with your own ambiguity. This means that our true being, our soul, is made up of opposing energies that spark and create the fire of life. Inside each one of us, there is both the divine and the diabolical, the sinner and the saint, the sacred and the profane, forbidden lust and unconditional love, the beatitude of Paradise and the dark night of the soul.

Being comfortable with your own ambiguity simply means being comfortable with these facts. To know that this is how it is, this is how God made us; this is what makes life interesting. A person who therefore exhibits both positive and negative qualities, who has strengths and weaknesses, is not flawed, but complete. When you accept this, when instead of always working on your weak points, you begin to release the guilt and shame that are the real culprits, you will become immensely attractive, for nothing is more desirable than this naturalness that radiates simple, unaffected humanity, blemishes and all. Being human has long been seen through tragic eyes, yet with a shift in perception being human is the essence of being lovable.

When you are comfortable with your own ambiguity, you will not be subject to behaviors that drive love away. These futile acts are a result of an inner dialogue that is constantly comparing you to an ideal that doesn't exist. This inner dialogue, based on the ego's fear, is constantly saying, 'I'm not good enough. I'm not thin enough. I'm not pretty or handsome enough. I'm not secure enough. I'm not rich enough.' Attractive people do not have this inner dialogue. Beautiful-looking people who have it going on are not really attractive, not to themselves.

Attractiveness also displays certain traits that make its possessor irresistible. Attractive people are not selective in their expression of love, not afraid to express it in any situation. Attractive people are not constantly looking for approval, which again comes from fear. Attractive people are never passive to the gestures of love that come our way in every moment of our lives. These gestures can take many forms: a smile from a stranger or a child, a twinkle in the eyes of someone you don't know, a warm handshake, a gentle squeeze, a hug, a compliment. Attractive people seize the moment to creatively respond with enthusiasm and gusto. And finally, attractive people are never comparing themselves to others or to an ideal.

To summarize, if you want to attract love and be attractive, then be natural. Be comfortable with your own ambiguities. Stop looking for approval. Don't be selective in your expression of love. Be lavish in your expression of love. Don't be passive. Respond creatively to every gesture of love. Don't compare yourself to others or to an ideal.

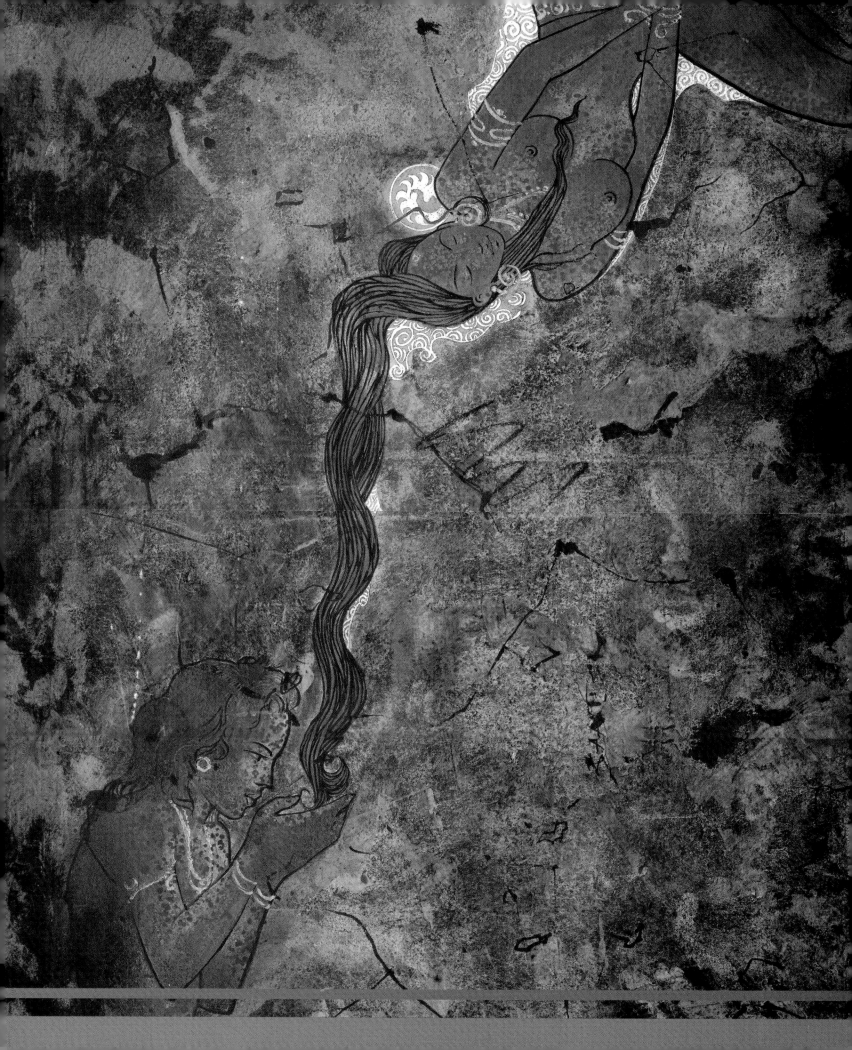

THE SECOND
STAGE OF LOVE:
INFATUATION

This law states that infatuation exists to open the door to a deeper, transcendent reality. Infatuation happens when the attraction between two people is so intense that it transports them beyond ordinary perception and the ordinary world becomes magical and enchanted.

Everyone has some experience of infatuation and the changes it brings. It takes you beyond the trivial and mundane; you rise above ordinary concerns (a glorious change that makes sensible people worry about how well you are coping with the rent or your next quarterly report). In spiritual terms, the infatuated vision of lovers is like the holy vision of saints. In the delirium of infatuation everything appears new. The release from old boundaries is what makes all things new. Lovers in this state worship each other. If infatuation is madness, sanity pales beside it. Infatuation is the second birth of innocence — and like a newborn child, the infatuated lover sees through eyes that make the world holy.

Although lovers speak of being reborn, in reality the source of newness is not a new person but a shift in perception. This shift moves from separation into unity. The infatuated lover sees the world as both immanent and transcendent, as though God has decided to live in the flowers and trees as well as in the beloved's body. But it is chiefly in the beloved's body that the holy seems to reside. Lovers may not know the meaning of immanence and transcendence, but then, words are not reality — they are only halting descriptions of reality. The immanent world is the ordinary world, apparent to our senses — material, changing, subject to time. The transcendent world is beyond the material — eternal and timeless. Infatuation opens the door to this transcendent reality.

We often hear more cynical observers saying of infatuated lovers, 'I wonder what they see in each other?' because outsiders see them as two ordinary people. And yet, it is the lovers, the infatuated ones, who have gone into a truer reality, because they have discovered the extraordinary in what everyone else sees as the ordinary. They see beyond the mask of appearance — a world that is unbounded, causeless, and timeless.

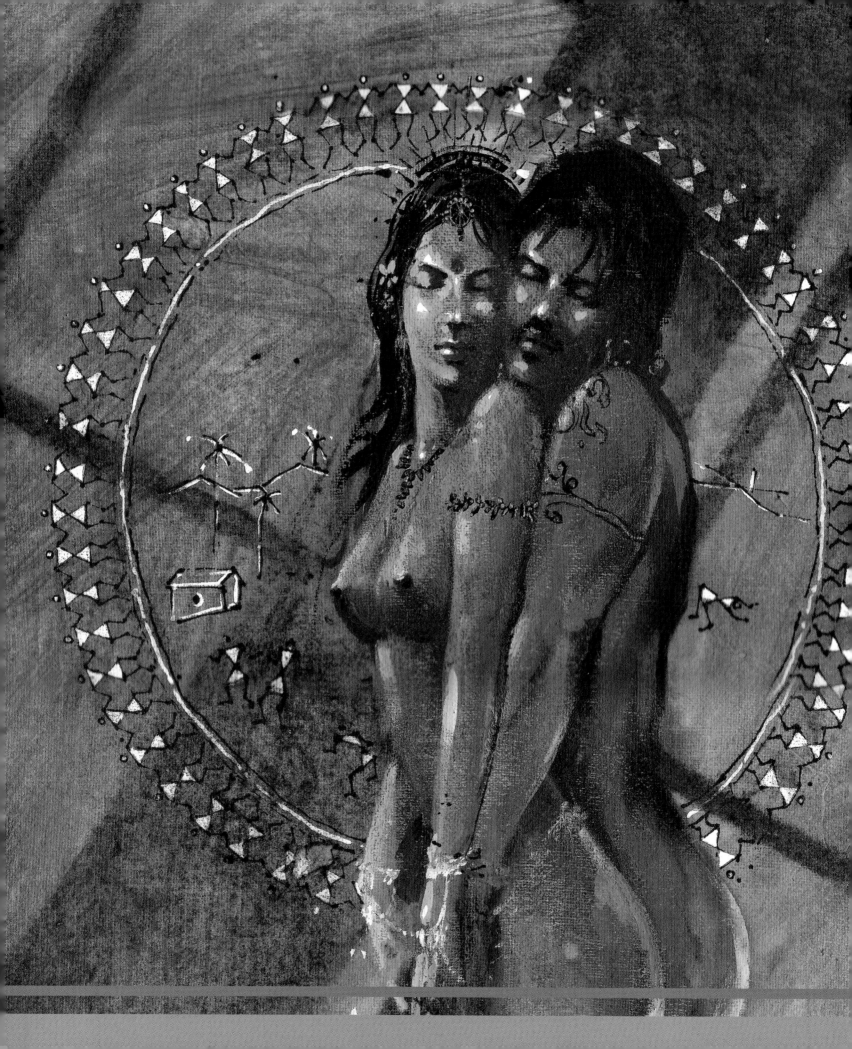

Rumi, the greatest of Sufi poets, says, 'Out beyond ideas of right doing and wrong doing, there is a field. I'll meet you there.' This 'going beyond' requires a new quality of awareness, something that has been called 'second attention'. First attention is ordinary awareness that allows you to see the obvious, the apparent, that which everybody else sees. Second attention is extraordinary awareness. It allows you to pierce the mask of appearance and go to the field of light, where everything magically connects with everything else. Some time or another we have all experienced this quality of awareness called second attention, if only when we have been carried away by art or music — or sex.

I would like to enumerate some examples of this hidden reality as it unexpectedly breaks through the mask of everyday life. Consider those moments, however fleeting, when you had any of the following experiences:

- You are in the midst of danger, yet you feel safe.
- There is turbulence and chaos and anxiety around you in your environment, but you feel deep peace inside.
- Somebody you know has an incurable illness, and they start to cure themselves, either permanently or for a time.
- In the noise and din of everyday existence you feel an unshakable inner silence.
- An inner voice speaks to you. This voice is nonverbal, pre-linguistic, intuitive. It guides you to make spontaneous and correct choices, weaving the web of your destiny.
- Sometimes when you look at people, you can see the light of their consciousness, the glow of their subtle body.
- A prayer gets answered; without explanation you feel cared for.
- You have a moment of wonder at the sight of a newborn child, or at the sheer fact of existence.
- You see yourself as a speck of awareness in the vast expanse of awareness, and you begin to expand until you become boundless, beyond the corridors of time and space.

These are all examples of the hidden reality that opens only to second attention. Infatuation opens the door to this hidden reality.

To summarize, if you want to experience the magical world of infatuated lovers, then look for the extraordinary in the ordinary. Learn to go beyond appearances. Look for the miraculous in everyday life. Culture the quality of awareness by second attention. Next time you see a flower, look at it again, keep gazing at it till you can see sunshine and rain and rainbows and earth and wind and fire and dust — until you can see the infinite void of space and the vast history of creation in that flower — and you can say with Rumi, 'Out beyond ideas of right doing and wrong doing, there is a field. I will meet you there.'

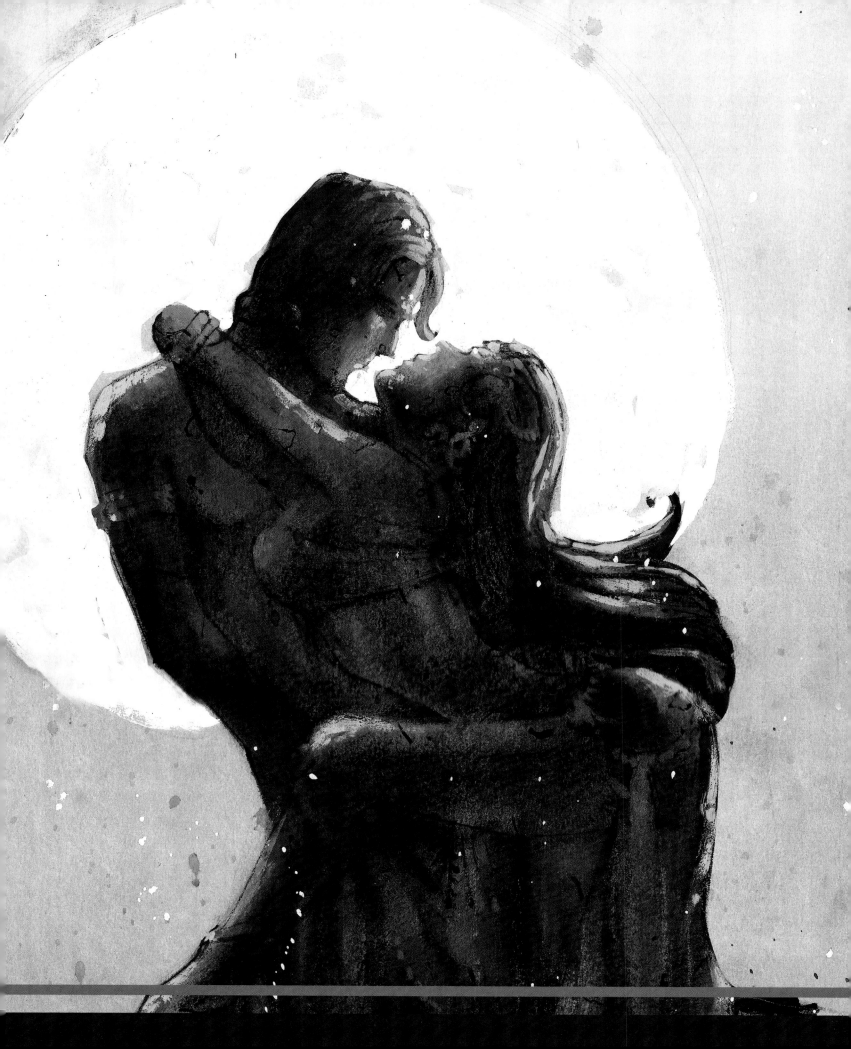

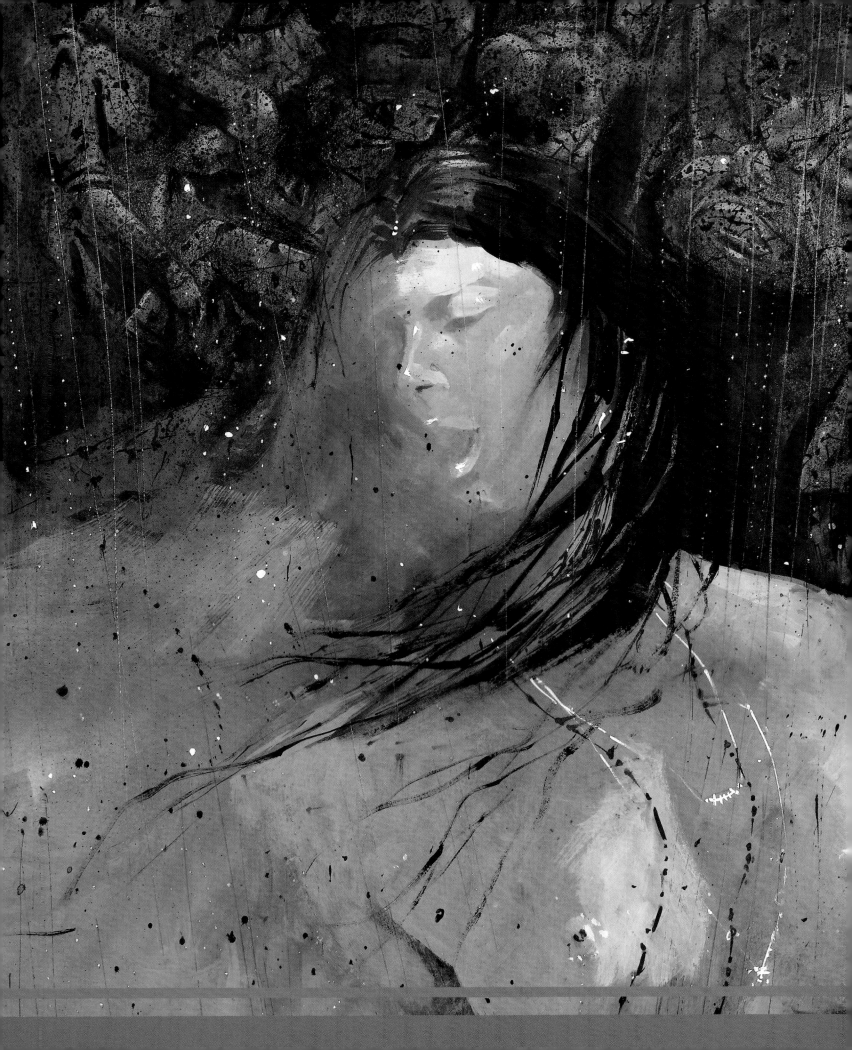

THE THIRD
STAGE OF LOVE:
COMMUNION

The Law of Communion says that communion is contact of soul with soul. Communion is the sharing of spirit. Therefore, communion is the basis of trust. In this stage, lovers move into the territory of the unknown, taking from each other what they did not possess alone. If their communion is deep enough, the perceptions of infatuation become real — you turn into the person you love.

Before communion occurs, the ego attempts to return and rear its ugly head. Ego wants to shatter the union of souls; it prefers the claims of I, me, and mine. 'We' can only be a temporary state. During this third phase, there is a battle between ego and love. This is essentially a battle for boundaries. If ego wins, then fear has projected itself from the past into the present through memory, and all the old boundaries are put back in place. 'I' is someone we all know very well from the past. 'We' is someone we are just beginning to know, and in that unknown quality a new future can unfold. The ego's resurfacing will interfere with communion and make it impossible to grow.

Communion is a phase where you are being tested. You will succeed if you and your beloved can dismantle your defenses together. Communion will fail if you build new defenses. So you must decide whether to borrow from one another and actually become what the other represents — the softness and tenderness and nurturing that a man finds in a woman is only borrowed unless you can teach yourself to develop these same qualities. A woman may benefit from the power, will, and strength of the man she loves, but that is not the same as having those qualities become your own. In communion you can become what you perceive, if your communion is deep enough.

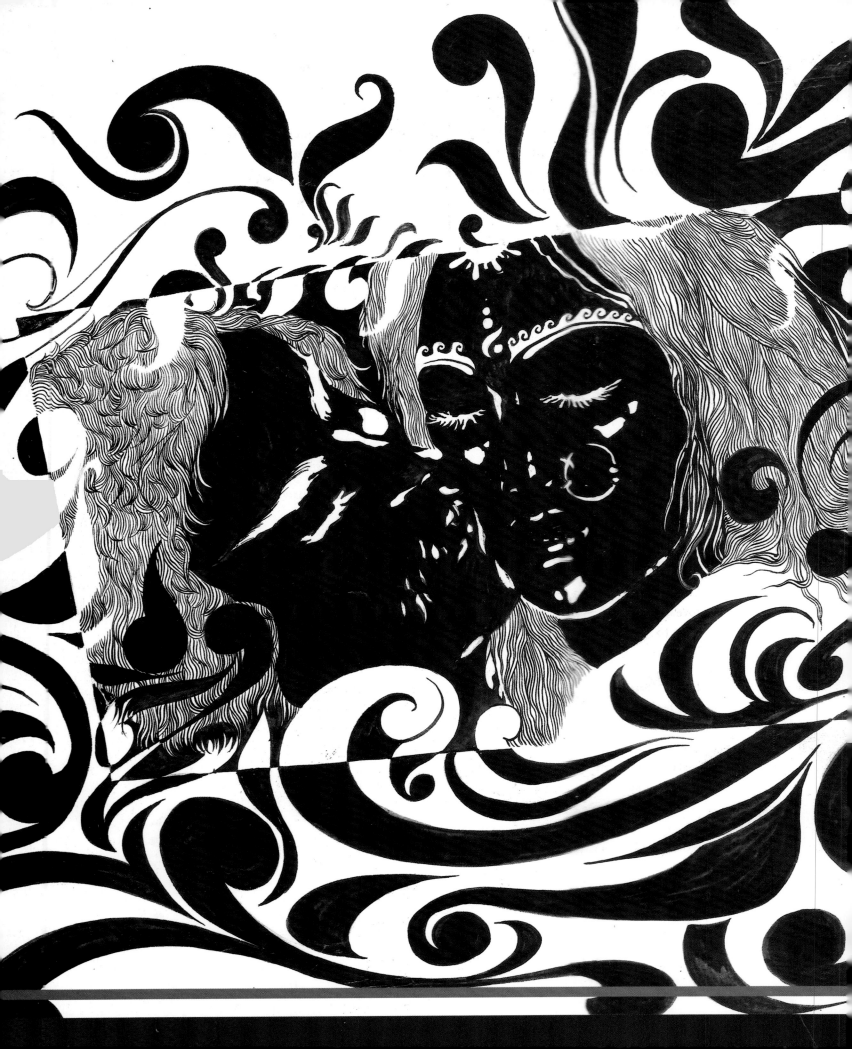

A problem that interferes with communion is the phenomenon of projection. Projection occurs when we attach our beliefs to another person. Frequently, we are unaware that we are projecting. If you display any of the following qualities, then you are participating in projection:

- You finish people's sentences for them.

- You act defensively even before being accused.

- You use verbal formulas, like 'He's the kind of person who gossips, or exaggerates, or tells lies'. In other words, you stereotype.

- You ask someone else's opinion, and then get angry if they disagree with you.

- You have a hard time reading people's faces.

- You frequently feel misunderstood.

- You see threat in the faces of authority figures, like policemen, or feel that your boss dislikes you, even though she has never said so.

- You believe that when your spouse or lover looks at another man or woman, sexual interest is being shown.

- You harbor extreme likes or dislikes about people you hardly know.

Getting rid of projection is critical if you want to be able to tell true love from false love, either as giver or receiver. Projection always hides deeper feelings that you don't want to look at. If you habitually defend yourself before being accused, you feel guilty. The guilt needs to be faced before you can stop the projection.

Projection is a way to psychologically turn the tables. As such, it masks the truth. If you feel that the man or woman you love is constantly looking at others with sexual interest, you are the one who cannot be trusted. If you think your boss secretly hates you, look at the possibility that you have hidden rage against authority. When you reclaim and bring home your feelings that you project onto others, you will feel liberated and feel less judgmental.

Besides stopping projection, we need to culture three necessary qualities for communion. These are:

- Equality
- Sensitivity
- Communication

Equality is the understanding that the spirit in everyone is equal. If I feel superior to you, my superiority is rooted in my self-image or ego.

Sensitivity is being able to sense what is going on inside another person. To be sensitive, you need to be able to accept the fact that emotions are complex, conflicting, confusing, and irrational. When we use expressions like, 'I don't understand why you feel this way,' or, 'I don't have the slightest idea what is going on with you,' then we have abandoned sensitivity. In order to be sensitive, we need to culture the following inner attitudes, which all have to do with empathy. Empathy is the ability to put yourself emotionally in someone else's shoes. An empathic person says:

- I don't need to be right all the time
- I don't need to be in control all the time
- I can ignore my needs for the time being

Finally, communion requires real communication. Social conventions and expectations interfere with true communication. Especially among men, conventions dictate that you are a strong person if you don't communicate your innermost feelings, and that you are weak if you do. Communication is impossible if you are unwilling or unable to expose yourself and communicate your vulnerabilities and your fears. Among women, communication is defeated when it becomes part of victimization. Poor me, you never talk to me anymore. This lament is a form of complaining, and all of us find it nearly impossible to open up to a complainer. The focus on self is so strong that emotionally no one else matters. So in demanding that the man talk about his emotions, the woman may really be saying, 'Do this because I need it. I don't really care what you say. I just want to feel better.'

True communication comes out of a joy in living with other souls, who are as interesting as you are yourself. Every soul is fascinating in the scheme of creation because at the soul level we are all exploring, each in a different way, the vastness of the unknown. When you realize this, communication becomes easy. You and your lover may have only a few things in common as personalities; you have eternity in common as souls.

To summarize, if you want to commune, identify the traits that you find attractive in your beloved. Instead of borrowing them, make a decision to become them. Identify your projective behavior. Stop projecting. Culture the qualities of equality, sensitivity and communication.

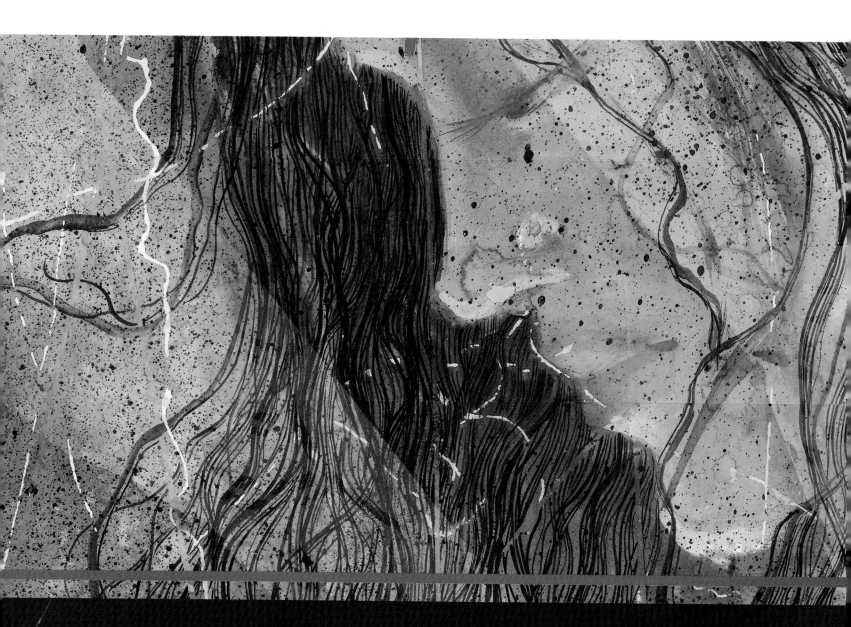

THE FOURTH STAGE OF LOVE: INTIMACY

The Law of Intimacy states that in true intimacy flesh merges with flesh, and spirit with spirit. In intimacy, sexual energy and spiritual energy are recognized as one. Sexual energy is seen as the creative energy of the universe. Intimacy is the union of one subtle body with another. Previously this was not complete. Attraction hints at sexual union and holds it out as a fantasy of pleasure. Infatuation brings the fantasy closer; communion makes it desirable as more than a brief encounter between two bodies. These three stages could conceivably take place in less than a day, even on first meeting.

Intimacy tests the fantasy by the actual blending of two separate people. This implies not just having sex but having it without boundaries, without turning orgasm into a selfish act. Every stage of love has its challenges. Intimacy is defeated when two people are in bed as two people; that is, they maintain their boundaries even when uniting. Intimacy succeeds when there is a release from boundaries. This happens on an energy level, which is why it becomes necessary to introduce the 'subtle body' as a new concept.

The subtle body dates from thousands of years ago. It has many names; the first, from Sanskrit, is Sukshma Sharir. Other traditions speak of the body of light, God's body, the Holy Ghost, the sacred breath. In all these cases one is speaking of the meeting point, the intersection that allows body and soul to make contact. In your subtle body you remain yourself, but at the same time you are more than yourself. You know more; you feel more. When you enter a room and sense that there is tension among people, when you know that someone has a good heart, when you divine that something unexpected is about to happen — all these shadowy bits of cognition come through your subtle body. It is also here that you determine whether to get sick or well, to be loved or unloved, to take a basically positive view of life or a negative one.

All this must be shared if you want to be intimate with another person. You cannot simply explain yourself in words, or even through action. Eventually your subtle body must come into contact with the other person's. In our society we don't use the phrase subtle body, but we do say 'give yourself away to someone else'. In wedding vows man and wife give themselves to each other. The reality behind this phrase exists at the level of the subtle body, where the only complete giving can take place.

In intimacy, we are so tuned in with the one we love that we feel their comfort, we feel their discomfort, we feel their emotions, we can read their thoughts, we can connect with their deepest intent. This bonding at all levels is also known as entrainment or coherence. There is a connection at all levels: sensual, sexual, emotional, and spiritual. The subtle body has channels to all three. In order to open these channels you need to get rid of certain socially programed ideas about physical relationships, sex, and spirituality. In this regard, I would like to offer the following insights regarding sexual energy and how to approach it spiritually when you feel ready for intimacy with someone you love.

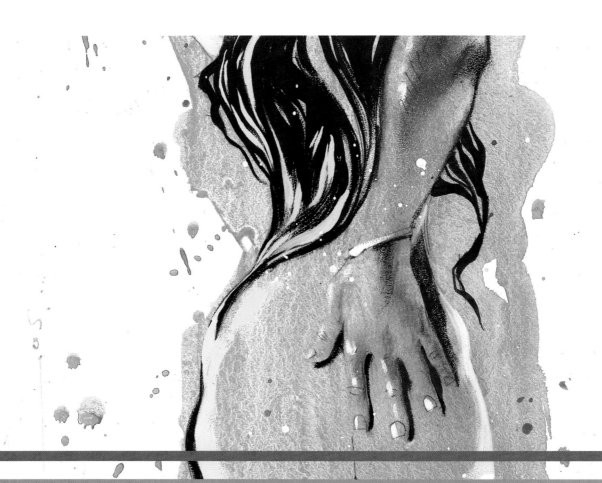

- Sexual energy is the primal and creative energy of the universe. All things that are alive come from sexual energy. In animals and other life forms, sexual energy expresses itself as biological creativity. In humans, sexual energy can be creative at all levels — physical, emotional, and spiritual. In any situation where we feel attraction, arousal, awakening, alertness, passion, interest, inspiration, excitement, creativity, or enthusiasm, in each of these situations, sexual energy is at work. Whenever we feel these states of awareness, we must put our attention on this energy that we are experiencing, nourishing it with our attention, experiencing it with joy and keeping it alive in our awareness.

- Sexual desire is sacred and chaste. The suppression of sexual energy is false, ugly, and unchaste.

- During sexual union, there is union between flesh and spirit through energy, an actual exchange at the subtle level.

- Bliss, carefreeness and playfulness are the essence of sexual energy in its most refined state.

- To improve your sexual experiences, get rid of your expectations. Expectations are always relics of the past; they occur primarily in three areas: performance, exemplified in the question, 'How am I doing?'; feeling, exemplified in the question, 'How am I feeling?'; and security, exemplified in the question, 'Do you love me?'

- In sex, as in all areas of life, resistance is born of fear. Fear is blocked energy. It is energy that says, 'If you experience me, you will be hurt or die.' All resistance is mental, because only the mind can decide what to experience and what to repress. It implies judgment against what is being felt. Sex becomes a problem when it gets mixed with feared emotions such as shame, guilt, and anger.

- Sexual intimacy is the road to the taste or experience of true freedom, because it is the one area of life in which we can become completely uninhibited and free.

- Sexual fulfillment occurs when the experience comes from playfulness instead of need. Frequently people bring their conflicts and needs into the sexual experience. When sex is used to fulfill needs, it leads to addiction. When sex comes from playfulness, the result is ecstasy.

- All problems related to sex, neurosis, deviancy, sexual misbehavior, violence, and abuse, can be traced to resistance, to suppression and repression, not to the sexual urges themselves. If we are allowed to discover our urges, desires, and emotions, without outside inhibition, they won't go to extremes. Extremism, in any form, is a reaction to repression, inhibition, and suppression. Aggression and violence are the shadow energies of fear and impotence.

- Sex is a means of escaping our little self or ego. It is many people's only experience of meditation.

- Meaningful sex has to be value-based. Values are personal. Each situation that has sexual energy in it involves the whole human being and their entire value system. My values may be different from yours, and I have no right to be the moral judge of anyone's values. It is important, however, to have core values, and respect them. Without values, we become spiritually bankrupt. Sexual experience will never cause problems and will always be joyful, if lovers share the same values.

These insights are touchstones of how much intimacy two people feel with each other. They aren't teachings out of sacred texts but real and personal experiences, repeated generation after generation. They are the legacy of being sexual creatures and at the same time having a soul. There is no timetable for having these insights. Two teenagers in the throes of puppy love may come closer to them than a married couple of fifty years who have grown bored with each other and experience love as a stale routine. As before, expectation is everything. If you expect to find a glory in intimacy, this is how it will unfold, at any age.

In summary, true intimacy is union between flesh and flesh, between subtle body and subtle body, between soul and soul. Sexual energy is sacred energy. When we have restored the sexual experience to the realm of the sacred, our world will be chaste and divine, holy and healed.

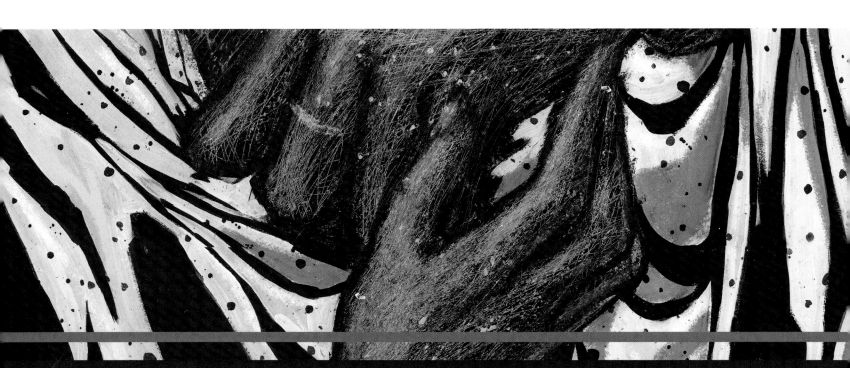

THE FIFTH STAGE OF LOVE: SURRENDER AND NON-ATTACHMENT

The Law of Surrender says that losing yourself in another person is the best way to find your true self. Surrender is the result of relinquishing the ego's last claims to separation. Surrender and non-attachment open the door to the miraculous, because miracles exist outside the realm of I, me, and mine. Many people mistakenly equate attachment with love when in fact attachment deprives us of love. Attachment goes into every situation asking, 'What can I get from this? What can I acquire for myself?' This impulse to possess comes from fear, and fear is the opposite of love. Attachment is always exclusive, and love is inclusive. Attachment is bondage, and love is freedom. Attachment is demanding, and love imposes no demands. Non-attachment is a state of freedom that preserves and increases your love for another. Attachment always seeks to control, and controlling people deeply fear abandonment. In true surrender, we never feel the need to control or cajole or convince or bully or manipulate or insist or beg or seduce. We know how to allow, and in that allowing, we invite love to move in and create miracles.

In the state of surrender and non-attachment, lovers display certain characteristics:

- ❧ They refuse to follow the impulses of anger and fear.

- ❧ They trust that the universe is on their side.

- ❧ They form their desires deep inside the heart and watch the higher self execute them.

- ❧ They believe they are enough as they are.

- ❧ They heed the tenderness and sweetness of their love for others.

- ❧ They put their full energy of love into every situation.

- ❧ They cultivate the peace of inner silence.

- ❧ They understand that nothing is ever lost, it is only transformed. The ingredients of life shift from one plane to another without distorting the exquisite balance of life.

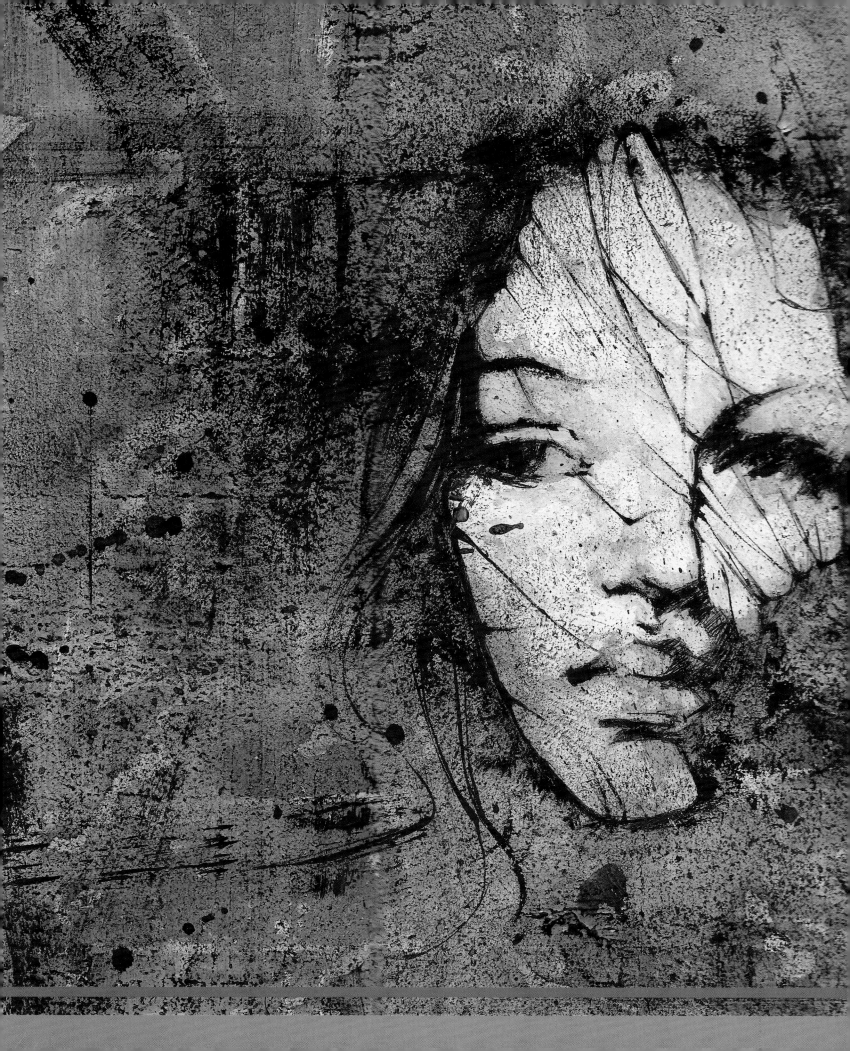

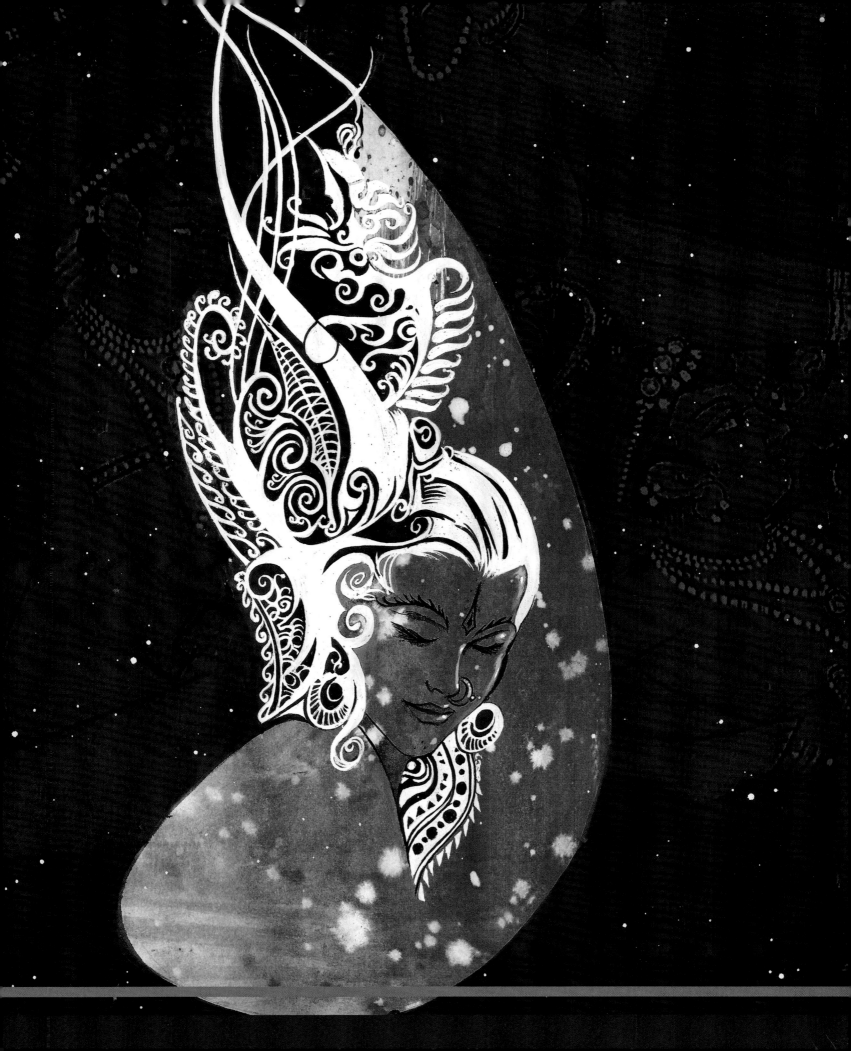

When anyone asks me how to make their relationship 'more spiritual', I keep this model in mind. I think surrender is very close to saintliness. In fact I can see no boundary between them. All the more sorrow that Western spirituality has ripped the two apart, making lovers and saints separate species in the human kingdom. If you are fortunate enough to follow the path of love until it reaches surrender, this stage will prove to you that this schism is false and damaging to love itself. Surrender to another person is surrender to spirit, because if you only give yourself as one person to another, the end result is a kind of slavery between two personalities, two egos. However, if you surrender in intimacy, where all is known and all is accepted, there is no question of personality. You are giving yourself to the true core of existence, which has traditionally been called the Self. In the *Brihadarunyaka Upanishad*, where a king and queen are discussing ideal love, the husband reminds the wife, 'Remember, you do not love me, you love me for the sake of the Self. You do not do anything for me, you do everything for the sake of the Self.' In this spirit, surrender to another is the most self-centered act you can perform; the secret is that your Self and your lover's are the same.

In summary, surrender brings to love the experience of the timeless. It brings the loss of ego. It brings an entry into the world of mysteries, which unfolds as the home of the beloved, but then is revealed as a place open to everyone who is capable of non-attachment.

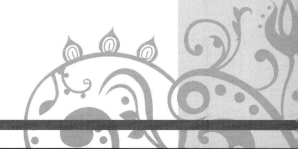

THE SIXTH
STAGE OF LOVE:
PASSION

The Law of Passion says that higher reality is experienced in the merging of the masculine and the feminine in one's own being. Passion for life and passion in love are the same thing. This is because life, in its essence, is love. Rumi once said, 'The most important thing in life is to become a passionate lover. If you have been a passionate lover in life, then you will be a lover in death, a lover in the tomb, a lover on the day of resurrection, a lover in Paradise, and a lover forever. But if you have not been a passionate lover in life, then count not your life as having been lived. On the day of reckoning, it will not be counted.'

Passion is not the same as physical hunger for someone else. Passion is real power. It will create anything you want, inspire you and your loved one to accomplish the impossible. It will move mountains. The mystery of passion is that although totally immaterial and subjective, it can conquer the material world and move objects. As in a dream, events unfold as your passion dictates they must. In the Vedic tradition the whole universe is a song of passion. It is the cosmic dance of Shiva, the masculine energy of creation, and Shakti, the feminine energy of creation. Human passion is kindled and sustained by these archetypal masculine and feminine energies as they interact with each other every day. In order to experience passion, there must be the merging of opposite energies; this merging brings a person into harmony with the soul, which merges all opposites:

- Loss and gain become the same, twinned aspects of fullness.

- Attraction and repulsion move together, depending on what is needed to come and go.

- Silence and activity join as the in-breath and out-breath of creation.

- Creation and destruction serve the same end, the constant unfolding of new forms of life.

Without using mythical labels, we can think of the universe operating this way, using opposite forces as twin aspects of creation. Thus it becomes possible to love death, because death is just another face of birth. It becomes possible to see yourself as both masculine and feminine, because both exist in everyone, whether they are male or female. In the Indian tradition the five masculine energies of Shiva are creation, protection, destruction, concealment, and revelation. In order to be alive — and aliveness is essentially the essence of passion — the spirit is constantly creating something, protecting something, destroying something, concealing something, and revealing something else.

These are totally necessary activities; without them life could not exist. Consider a baby of two years old. New cells are constantly being created, new abilities acquired. These are protected — that is, sustained — in memory so that the child can continue to develop. At the same time, infantile behavior is departing or being destroyed; we don't tend to notice this as much because our eyes are fascinated by all the new things a baby is turning into. Concealed from view, but just as real, are parts of the genetic program to come in the future, such as the replacement of baby teeth and the arrival of puberty. Revelation comes in the form of delighted perception unfolding in the baby's awareness, a sense of a new world being born that has surprising things to reveal around every corner.

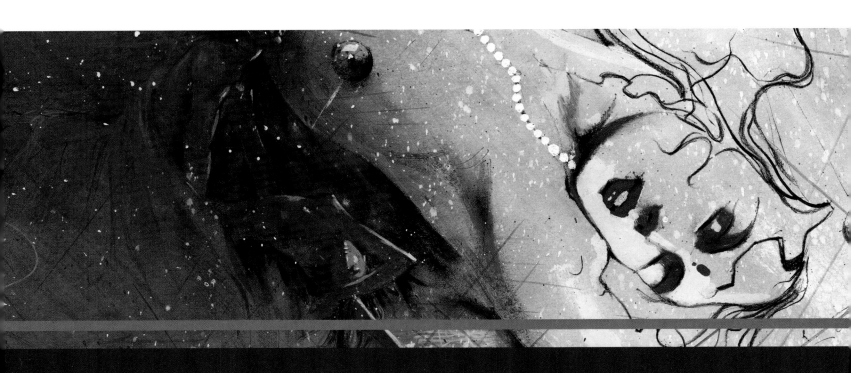

Can you extend these five processes to your own life? If they have stopped in one way or another, you are stifling a cosmic energy, a divine force. In adults the loss of passion is marked through three qualities:

- Creation is lost when nothing new seems to happen anymore.
- Protection turns into a smothering desire to keep the past in place, to live out of habit and conditioning.
- Revelation becomes impossible because the doors of perception are closed; one sees only the mundane world colored by shadows from the past.

Passion is just another name for keeping all five divine energies alive. As we move through life, we must constantly ask ourselves, 'What am I creating? What am I protecting? What habits or toxicities in my life must I get rid of in order to renew myself? What will I reveal about my intent to those around me? How can I best find the spirit concealed within me?'

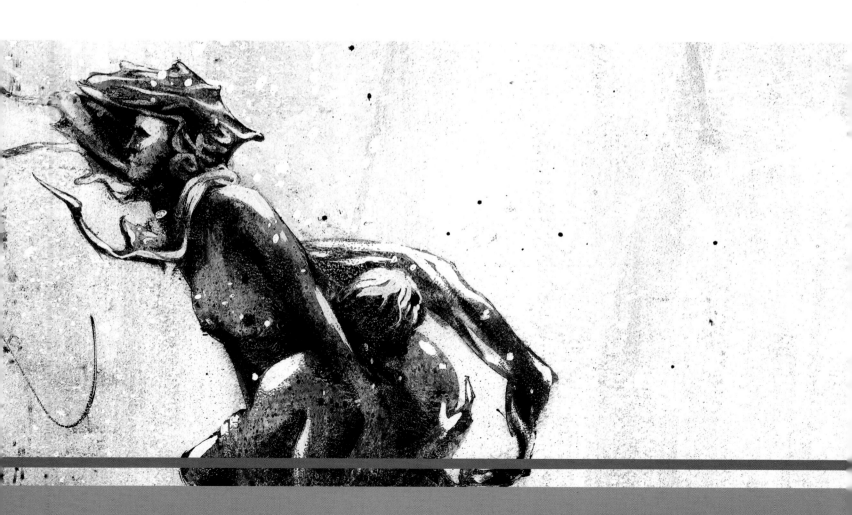

In India the five feminine energies, sometimes lumped together simply as Shakti, or feminine power, are:

- Pure consciousness. This is uncreated power, inherent in pure consciousness or Chitta Shakti, where there is no thought or desire. The affirmation or mantra that evokes this Shakti is 'I am.'

- Bliss, or Ananda Shakti. This is the knowingness that bliss is my essential state, that I need not do anything or require anything to experience it. The mantra or affirmation to evoke this Shakti is 'I am bliss.'

- Pure intent, the Shakti inherent in desire, an intent that wants to create joy and fulfillment. The mantra or affirmation to evoke this Shakti is 'I intend or I desire.'

- Pure knowingness beyond rationality. This is the intuition that allows us to do the right thing at the right time, because our intent has tapped into the cosmic mind. The mantra or affirmation to evoke the Shakti is 'I know.'

- The power of pure action, Kriya Shakti. Kriya is the name for an action which is independent of belief, expectations, interpretations, memory, or fear. It is the action that is rooted in awareness and creativity. The affirmation to evoke this Shakti is 'I act.'

If these five masculine and five feminine energies are kept lively in our own awareness, then we begin to experience passion. In addition to these energies on the spiritual level, there are five masculine and feminine energies on the emotional level. The five masculine energies on the emotional level are courage, discipline, decisiveness, strength, and chivalry. On the feminine side the five energies on the emotional level are beauty, intuition, nurturing, affection, and tenderness.

In summary, passion is the merging of the masculine and feminine forces in our own beings. Passion in life and passion in love keep the fire of life alive and spark the birth of creation.

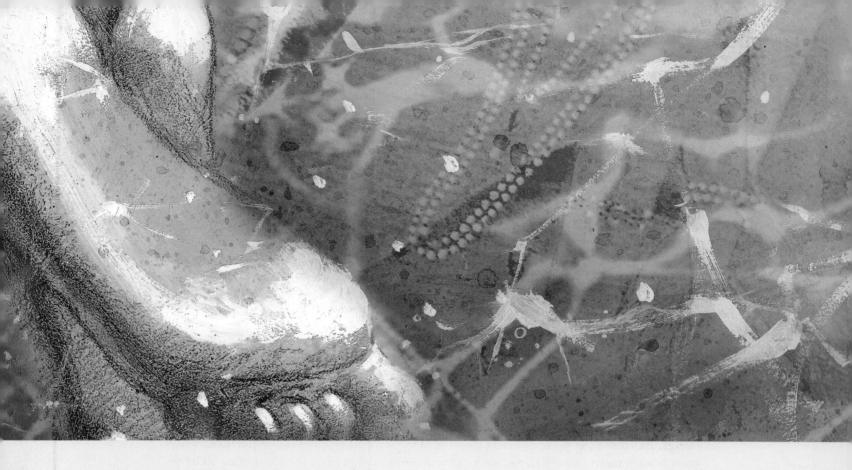

THE SEVENTH
STAGE OF LOVE:
ECSTASY

The Law of Ecstasy says that ecstasy is our original state. This is where we come from, the Garden of Eden, the state of grace to which we shall one day return. Ecstasy is the final stage of intimacy with spirit that flows through love. Here, even exuberance, joy, delight, and satisfaction are seen as shadows of the Real, whose ecstasy is like a master vibration that everything in nature is trembling to express.

We cannot speak anymore of a higher and lower self. In ecstasy, there is a merging of the individual ego with the cosmic ego, and the spontaneous knowing, 'I am that, you are that, all this is that, and that alone is' — *Tat twam asi*. In this stage, personal love and universal love, human love and divine love merge to become pure love, unconditional and simple. There are three ingredients to this divine state:

Physical ecstasy. Physical ecstasy comes from the world of our senses. This happens when we have life-centered, present-moment awareness and our senses are alive to every nuance of touch, sound, sight, taste, and smell. When we give full attention to every texture and flavor of life and to love in every aspect of our being, our life becomes sensuous and we realize that God created a sensuous universe, a recreational universe to nourish our spirit. We take delight in touching and being touched, feasting our eyes on the beauty of the physical body and the physical world, feeling nourished in every pore of our being. Through our senses we find the doorway to God.

Myth and archetype. In ordinary perception, we see ourselves in unmythic terms. Our natural ecstatic state is overshadowed by trivial concerns and mundane activity. The reality, however, is that beneath the turmoil of our daily activity, our real, our unconscious motivations dwell in the mythical world. Inside us are primal gods and primal goddesses. We know this without knowing it insofar as we obey our mythic drives without bringing them into conscious awareness. When we do magnificent things, like building great cathedrals or creating great art or science, or partake in any great achievement, we are allowing the primal gods and goddesses to be born. Striving to succeed in big business partakes of the heroic journey as much as the Argonauts seeking the golden fleece. Climbing Everest is driven by the same ambition, to reach the abode of gods, as with Icarus flying toward the sun. In mythic terms, ecstasy is a sacred journey into the underworld, heroically portrayed in countless versions from Persephone's abduction by Pluto to Orpheus seeking his bride among the shades of Hades. In ancient Greece, the worship of Dionysius was not about excess but about attaining divine ecstasy. When we lose mythology, we become spiritually impoverished and languish into dullness. Our kids join street gangs because of this mythical need to express the magnificence of their own being. Gangs, though misguided, have initiation rites and rituals, leadership and imagination, all active ingredients of a life-sustaining mythology. It is for the same reason that adults join cults. Our modern society has been mythically deprived. Perhaps with a new age of awareness, and the opening up of new frontiers through space technology, we will start a new mythical journey. Beyond the seas of space lies the new raw material for our imagination. In both inner and outer space are the ingredients of a new mythology. Mystery, adventure, wonder, imagination, new challenges; all these await us and with them perhaps the coming of an age such as Homer never dreamed of.

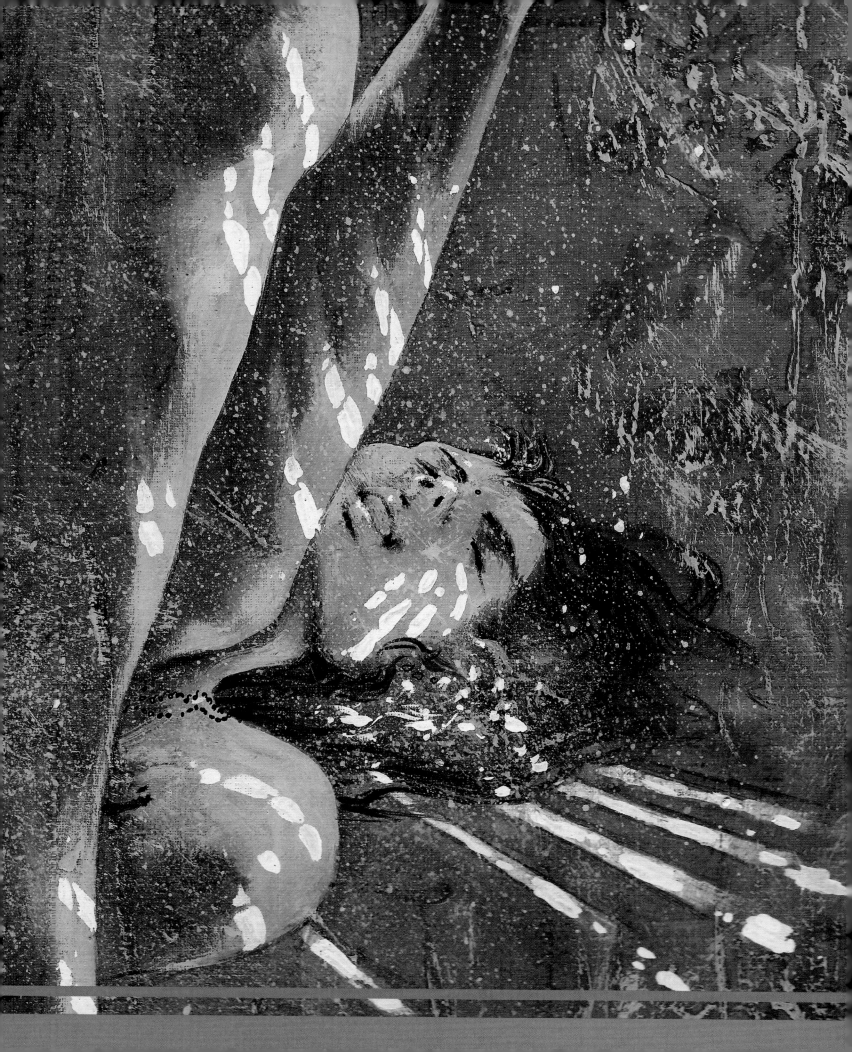

Spiritual ecstasy. Spiritual ecstasy is a face-to-face meeting with Spirit or God. Spiritual ecstasy is inclusive of physical and mythical ecstasy, but must also derive from the devotion (Bhakti) or worship of the true seeker who says to God, 'My sweet Lord, I only want to see you, Lord, it takes so long, but I want to see your face, my sweet God.' It is the ecstasy of yearning, and yearning is the mask of divine ecstasy that Rumi expresses so well.

So, when we have physical, mythical and sacred ecstasy, we have arrived where we started from. We are holy and we are healed.

To summarize, ecstasy is a primordial energy state. To experience ecstasy, we must satisfy our physical, sensual, mythical, and spiritual needs. In the return of ecstasy we can say with Solomon:

> *You split me, and tore my heart open. You filled me with love. You poured your spirit into mine. I knew you as I know myself. My eyes are radiant with your light. My ears delight in your music. My nostrils are filled with your fragrance. My face is covered with your dew. You have made all things new. You have made me see all things shining. You have granted me perfect ease. I have become like Paradise.*

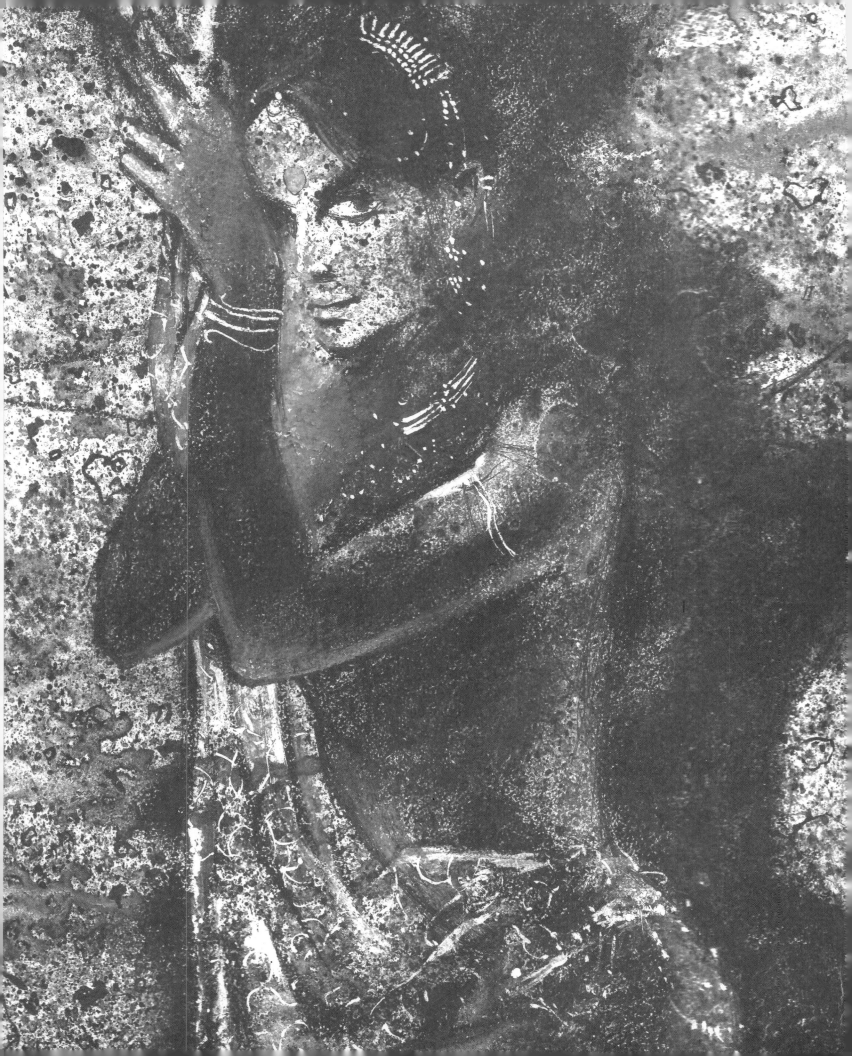